Gillian Hawthorne
(Editor)

Diabetes Care
for the Older Patient

A Practical Handbook

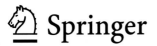 Springer

Editor
Gillian Hawthorne, MBBCH.,
BAO., Ph.D., FRCP (London)
Newcastle Diabetes Centre
The Newcastle upon Tyne
Hospitals, NHS Foundation Trust
Campus for Ageing and Vitality
Newcastle upon Tyne
UK

ISBN 978-0-85729-460-9   e-ISBN 978-0-85729-461-6
DOI 10.1007/978-0-85729-461-6
Springer London Dordrecht Heidelberg New York

A catalogue record for this book is available from the British Library

Library of Congress Control Number: 2011933719

Cover design: eStudioCalamar, Figueres/Berlin

Printed on acid-free paper

Springer is part of Springer Science+Business Media (www.springer.com)

For Jim, Andrew, Robert and Joanna

Foreword: Diabetes in the Elderly

The world is in the grip of a pandemic of type 2 diabetes. Numbers of people affected are rising inexorably with current numbers estimated at 346 million and almost 500 million more at high risk. It is occurring in young people as well as adults and prevalence rises sharply in the elderly. Type 2 diabetes is not a benign disorder: it leads to the specific microvascular complications of diabetes-retinopathy, renal damage and neuropathy and is a major risk factor for macrovascular disease including ischaemic heart disease, stroke and peripheral vascular disease. All of the latter are more common than in the non-diabetic population and peripheral vascular disease results in the risk of foot ulcers and amputations.

The specific molecular mechanisms underlying type 2 diabetes remain elusive. It is more common in those with a family history of the disorder and certain ethnic groups appear to be at particular risk. It is also more common in the elderly. The major associations are, however, with lifestyle. The weight of the population is rising dramatically and in parallel physical activity is decreasing. Both of these are associated with insulin resistance and this leads to type 2 diabetes in those with inadequate insulin secretory reserve. Obviously the best approach is prevention but outside specific research studies countries have singularly failed to make the changes required to decrease obesity and increase physical activity. In the meantime, it is key that people who already have diabetes receive the care and attention required to prevent complications.

Older people require particular attention. Diabetes is often not diagnosed and largely ignored. The number of affected older people is rising rapidly, many have multiple co-morbidities. Even when recognised the seriousness of diabetes in this age group is often underestimated. In particular there are problems in residential care where staff are often unskilled and lack knowledge of diabetes. Poorly controlled blood glucose levels are associated with increased risk of infection, poor wound healing, nocturia dehydration – all of which can present particular problems in the elderly. A further poorly recognised problem is the common occurrence of depression in people with type 2 diabetes.

The present volume could not be more timely. It not only draws attention to the importance of type 2 diabetes in a major underserved section of the community but also gives practical guidance on the management of diabetes and its associated problems, specifically in the elderly. It will be of particular help to carers of older people with diabetes and all those involved in their day-to-day care. It fills a large gap and hopefully will help improve care in this growing part of our community.

K.G.M.M. Alberti
Chair, Diabetes UK
Senior Research Investigator
Imperial College, London

Preface

Diabetes mellitus has reached epidemic proportions and more than half of all people with diabetes in the UK are aged 60 years and over. So the combination of an ageing population with a diabetes epidemic means that older people with diabetes are coping with problems related to the management and treatment of diabetes and at the same time they are also facing an additional burden related to ageing and associated co-morbidities. The complexities of their care are often overlooked.

This book aims to provide a practical guide to managing diabetes in older people for those healthcare professionals on the front line. Most clinical evidence used to inform treatment and management of diabetes is derived from randomised controlled trials but the evidence from these trials is often not applicable to older people as they are usually excluded from clinical trial populations. Clinical targets derived from these trials and set for the management of an older individual may be inappropriate in the presence of significant co-morbidity.

This older group has particular problems; the physiology of ageing changes their response to therapy and other problems such as dementia, depression and frailty have a significant impact on the treatment and management of their diabetes. Chapters on these topics review current research evidence of the impact and interaction of diabetes and discuss management of these problems. Practical guidance on the management of cardiovascular risk factors and glucose targets is included. A major complication of therapy, hypoglycaemia, may not be readily recognised in older people and a chapter is devoted to exploring avoidance and recognition of this.

Finally the last section looks at the delivery of care. Carers are closely involved in the day to day living of older people with diabetes. Practical guidance, information and support for carers are described. The general practitioner is key to managing all of this and the last chapter highlights some of the daily challenges that general practitioners need to address when trying to provide high-quality care.

There is no doubt that the complexities of diabetes care associated with ageing will continue to dominate clinical practice in the foreseeable future. I hope this book is a valuable aid and an enjoyable read for those healthcare professionals working in this field.

Contents

List of Contributors

Terry J. Aspray, M.B.B.S., M.D., FRCP, FRCP (Edin)
Bone Clinic, Freeman Hospital,
Newcastle upon Tyne, UK and
Institute for Ageing and Health, Newcastle University,
Newcastle upon Tyne, UK

Mima Cattan, Ph.D., M.Sc., B.Sc. (Hons)
School of Health, Community and Education Studies,
Northumbria University, Newcastle upon Tyne, UK

Tom Coulthard, MCChB, M.Sc., MRCGP
General Practitioner, Heaton Medical Centre,
Newcastle upon Tyne, UK

Simon C.M. Croxson, M.D., FRCP
Department of Medicine for the Elderly,
University Hospitals Bristol NHS Foundation Trust,
Bristol Royal Infirmary, Bristol, UK

Gillian Hawthorne, MBBCH., BAO., Ph.D., FRCP (London)
Newcastle Diabetes Centre, The Newcastle upon Tyne
Hospitals, NHS Foundation Trust, Campus for Ageing and
Vitality, Newcastle upon Tyne, UK

Louise Hayes, B.A. (Hons), M.Sc., Ph.D.,
Institute of Health and Society, Newcastle University,
Newcastle upon Tyne, UK

Gemma M. Smith, M.B.B.S., MRCP (Edin)
Department of Elderly Care,
Sunderland Royal Hospital, Sunderland, UK

**Mark W.J. Strachan, B.Sc. (Hons),
MBChB (Hons), M.D., FRCP (Edin)**
Metabolic Unit, Western General Hospital, Edinburgh, UK

Alan J. Thomas, MRCPsych, Ph.D.,
Wolfson Research Centre, Institute for Ageing and Health,
Newcastle University, Newcastle upon Tyne, UK

Nigel C. Unwin, B.A., M.Sc., DM, FRCP, FFPH
Public Health and Epidemiology, Faculty of Medical
Sciences, University of the West Indies, Cave Hill, Barbados

Akshya Vasudev, M.B.B.S., M.D., MRCPsych, PG Cert Med Ed
Department of Geriatric Psychiatry,
University of Western Ontario and Lawson
Research Institute, London, ON, Canada

Alison J. Yarnall, M.B.B.S. (Hons), MRCP
Clinical Ageing Research Unit,
University of Newcastle upon Tyne,
Newcastle upon Tyne, UK

Chapter 1
The Epidemiology of Diabetes in Older People

Louise Hayes and Nigel C. Unwin

Background

The prevalence of diabetes increases into older age in both men and women [1] (Fig. 1.1). This is of considerable concern in the context of the UK's ageing population. Diabetes is a major health problem in the elderly, contributing to both increased morbidity and mortality, and increasing substantially the demand an elderly population makes on the health care system [2]. Estimates of total (known and undiagnosed) diabetes for England suggest that 14.3% (with an uncertainty range of 10.6–19.2%) of men and women aged 55–74 years have diabetes, rising to 16.5% (12.3–22.0%) in those aged over 75 years [3]. Indeed it is estimated that more than half of all people with diabetes in the UK are aged 60 years or over [4].

As the elderly population increases as a proportion of the total population the prevalence and health consequences of diabetes in the elderly are of increasing importance. Recent estimates suggest that by 2034 almost a quarter of the UK population, in excess of 15 million individuals, will be aged over 65 years [5]. A conservative estimate based on the current estimate of diabetes prevalence of 14.3% in the 55–74 year

L. Hayes (✉)
Institute of Health and Society, Newcastle University,
Baddiley-Clark Building, Richardson Road, NE2 4AX
Newcastle upon Tyne, UK

G. Hawthorne (ed.), *Diabetes Care for the Older Patient*,
DOI 10.1007/978-0-85729-461-6_1,
© Springer-Verlag London Limited 2012

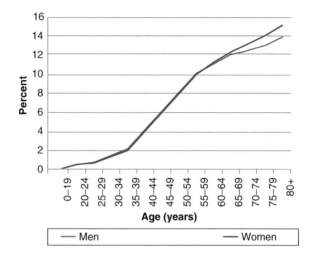

FIGURE 1.1 Global diabetes prevalence by age and sex for 2000 (adapted from [4])

age-group [3] would mean that in excess of 2,145,000 people aged over 65 years will be living with diabetes by 2034. The actual figure is likely to be higher as trends in diabetes prevalence and risk factors for type 2 diabetes are upward.

This chapter reviews the current and likely future epidemiology of diabetes in the elderly in the UK, the association of diabetes in the elderly with morbidity and mortality and discusses the diagnosis of diabetes in the elderly.

'Elderly' here is used to refer to the proportion of the population that is aged 60 years and over, although due to the availability of data, some information is presented for those aged 65 years and over.

The Elderly Population of the UK – Size and Trends

It is clear that the UK population, like populations the world over, is ageing. Since the middle of the twentieth century the proportion of the UK population aged 60 years and older has

TABLE 1.1 The elderly population in the UK by year

Age		1951	2001	2031
≥60 years	Millions	7.9	12.2	19.4
	% total population	15.7%	20.8%	30.0%
≥65 years	Millions	5.5	9.3	15.2
	% total population	10.9%	15.9%	23.5%

Adapted from [6]

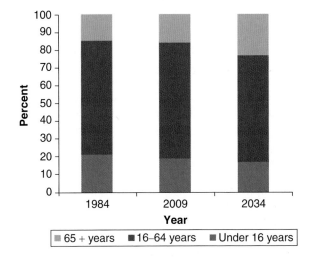

FIGURE 1.2 The UK's ageing population (adapted from [5])

increased from under 16% in 1951 to almost 21% in 2001. It is predicted that by 2031 almost a third of the UK population will be aged 60 years and older (Table 1.1) [6]. The increase in the proportion aged 65 years and older is even more marked, from under 11% in 1951 to a predicted 23.5% in 2031.

In the 25 years between 1984 and 2009 the population aged 65 years and over increased by 1.7 million individuals, at the same time as the population aged under 16 years was decreasing. It is anticipated that by 2034 the proportion of the population aged over 65 years will be greater than that aged under 16 years (23% compared to 18%) (Fig. 1.2) [5].

Not only will the proportion of elderly in the UK population continue to increase, but the ethnic composition of the elderly will change. There will be an increasing proportion from Black and Asian groups, who are known to be at greater risk of diabetes than the White population. It is estimated that as a proportion of those aged 60 years and older in the UK the Asian population will increase from 1.6% in 2001 to 2.7% in 2020 and the Black population from 1.0% to 1.3% [7].

The Prevalence of Diabetes in the Elderly in the UK

The prevalence of known, or diagnosed, diabetes in the elderly in the four countries of the UK by age-group and sex is shown in Fig. 1.3. A similar pattern in diabetes prevalence is seen in each of the four countries, with prevalence being higher in men than women (with the exception of the 65–74 year age-group in Northern Ireland) and a general increase in prevalence apparent with age, but with a plateau or decline in the oldest age-group. Overall the prevalence in

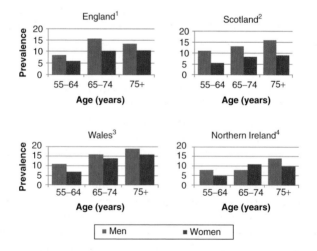

FIGURE 1.3 Prevalence of diagnosed diabetes in four UK countries

men aged 65 years and older is around 14% and in women in this age-group is approximately 10%.

Other studies from the UK have reported a prevalence of known diabetes in elderly White populations of between 3% and 14%. The Southall Diabetes Survey and the Coventry Diabetes Study reported a prevalence of diabetes in those aged 65 years and older of around 3% [1, 8] and a GP practice-based study conducted in Melton Mowbray in 1987 reported a prevalence in the same age-group of 6% [9]. In a GP practice-based study in Newcastle-upon-Tyne the prevalence of known diabetes in those aged 60 years and older was 7.4% [10], and in the British Regional Heart Study in 2005, a prevalence of 10.9% was reported in those aged 65–69 years, rising to 14.2% in those aged 75–79 years [11]. The wide range in the reported prevalence of known diabetes in the elderly is likely attributable to both real increases over time in the incidence of diabetes in this age-group, as a result of increased prevalence of obesity and related risk factors, and to improvements in case ascertainment.

Both the incidence and prevalence of diabetes are increasing globally and this is largely attributed to changes in lifestyle as well as demographic change [12]. Data from the Health Survey for England over the period 1994–2006 show that the prevalence of diagnosed diabetes in those aged 65 years and older has increased consistently in both men and women in England from below 6% to almost 16% and from 5% to over 10% in men and women respectively aged 65–74 years in this period and from 7% to 13% and from 5% to almost 11% in men and women aged 75 years and older. Analysis of data from over 7,000 men in the British Regional Heart Survey has shown that the prevalence of diabetes has increased substantially, by approximately 7% each year, in middle-aged and elderly men over the last quarter of a century in the UK [11]. Furthermore, evidence of an acceleration in the rate of increase is apparent. Between 1979 and 1984 the prevalence increased by 4% each year, but in the last 5 years for which data were available, this increase had risen to over 10% annually [11]. The available evidence suggests that the prevalence of diagnosed diabetes in the elderly has doubled over the last 15–20 years.

It should be noted that these figures are for diagnosed diabetes only. A substantial proportion of diabetes that is undiagnosed exists. It has been estimated that a little over a quarter of people with diabetes are currently undiagnosed [13]. A recent diabetes screening study in a single GP practice in Newcastle upon Tyne found that 37% of 584 community dwelling individuals aged 60 years and older identified with diabetes at screening on the basis of an oral glucose tolerance test (OGTT) were previously undiagnosed [10]. A previous study undertaken between 1986 and 1989 in Coventry, which included a larger sample of 1,100 individuals aged 65 years and older reported a much higher proportion of undiagnosed diabetes, particularly in the European origin population [1]. In the Coventry Diabetes Study it was found that 70% of European origin women and 58% of European origin men with diabetes diagnosed by OGTT at screening were previously undiagnosed. In contrast, over 50% of the South Asian origin population with diabetes had been previously diagnosed. The reason for higher previous diagnosis in the South Asians in this study is unclear, but it has been hypothesised that it is likely to be attributable to an earlier age at onset of diabetes in these individuals [1]. In contrast, in a study of over 1,000 very elderly individuals (The Newcastle 85+ Cohort Study) undiagnosed diabetes was found to be relatively low at approximately 14% [14]. The substantially higher proportion of undiagnosed diabetes reported in the Coventry Diabetes Study than in the more recent studies and that estimated by the Association of Public Health Observatories (APHO) Diabetes Prevalence model may reflect improvements in case ascertainment over recent years [15].

Where screening for diabetes has been conducted among the elderly residents of care homes in the UK a total (including known and diabetes newly diagnosed at screening) prevalence of approximately 25% has been reported [16, 17].

Some studies have reported that a plateau or decrease in diabetes prevalence occurs at around the age of 80–85 years.

The Medical Research Council (MRC) trial of assessment and management of older people in the community reported a lower prevalence of diabetes in men and women aged 85–89 years of 6.8% compared to 8.3% in those aged 75–79 years [2]. There is some evidence that the occurrence of new cases of diabetes declines in the very elderly (aged 80 years and above) [18]. It is unclear to what extent any reported decline in incidence or prevalence of diabetes reflects the method used to identify or diagnose individuals with diabetes [19]. There is evidence from some studies of a higher rate of undiagnosed diabetes in older individuals. For example, the Newcastle-upon-Tyne screening study found that 37% of all individuals aged 60 years and older with diabetes were previously undiagnosed, but a higher proportion (43%) of those aged 75 years and older was undiagnosed.

Method of Diagnosis and Prevalence of Diabetes in the Elderly

Not all studies have found a high rate of undiagnosed diabetes in the most elderly or a decline in diabetes incidence and prevalence in this group. As reported above, the rate of undiagnosed diabetes in the Newcastle 85+ Study was relatively low (approximately 14%) on the basis of a fasting blood glucose of 7.0 mmol/l or greater [14]. It is possible that the method used to identify previously undiagnosed diabetes (fasting blood glucose) identified fewer individuals than would have been identified if a post-glucose challenge measure had been used [16]. The use of fasting blood glucose to diagnose diabetes in elderly care home residents results in fewer diagnoses being made than if post-prandial glucose is used [16]. Similarly if HbA_{1c} is used diagnostically a smaller proportion of undiagnosed diabetes may be found. In the Newcastle screening study in men and women aged 60 years and older previously undiagnosed diabetes was 28% when an HbA_{1c} of 6.5% [48 mmol/mol] or greater was used for diagnosis, rather than the 37% when using OGTT for diagnosis.

The MRC trial reported a lower prevalence of diabetes in the very elderly (those aged 85 years and older), but, although a random glucose measurement >11.1 mmol/l was considered diagnostic, the diagnosis of diabetes was largely self-reported or extracted from medical records. Other studies have reported conflicting results. In a 20 year follow-up of almost 3,000 adults recruited to the Whickham Survey of diabetes and lipid disorders it was found that diabetes incidence continued to rise even in the most elderly age-groups [20].

If it is accepted that a decline in diabetes incidence occurs in the very elderly the reason for this has not been elucidated but a likely explanation is that those who would be susceptible to developing diabetes die from other causes before onset or diagnosis of diabetes occurs.

The Distribution of Diabetes in the Elderly by Ethnicity

The prevalence of diabetes is also patterned by ethnicity. It has been established that certain ethnic groups, including individuals of South Asian and Black African or Caribbean ancestry experience higher rates of diabetes than those of European or Chinese ancestry. The Southall Diabetes Survey, carried out in the 1980s, reported an age-adjusted prevalence of known diabetes in South Asians that was 3.8 times that found in Europeans [8]. Data collected in the Health Survey for England in 2004 showed that the prevalence of diagnosed diabetes in Black Caribbean and Indian men was more than double that of the general population [21]. The APHO diabetes model estimates that total diabetes prevalence in the adult South Asian population in England is 14% and that in adults of Black ethnicity is almost 10% compared to just under 7% for those of White, mixed or other ethnic group [3]. The higher diabetes prevalence found in South Asians compared to Europeans is partly attributable to an earlier onset of diabetes in South Asians. In the Southall Diabetes Survey, for example, the difference in prevalence between South Asians and Europeans was most marked in those aged 40–64 years, when a five-fold excess was reported in South Asians [8]. Despite a reduction in the magnitude of the difference in prevalence in the elderly, an excess of diabetes in elderly South Asians compared to Europeans has been reported. In the Southall Diabetes Survey in those aged 75 years and older diabetes prevalence in South Asians was 2.5 times that in Europeans. In the Coventry Diabetes Study a greater excess of known diabetes in elderly South Asians compared to Europeans was reported. Overall for those aged 65 years and over known diabetes prevalence was 5.5 times higher in South Asian men than in European men (17.6% compared to 3.2%) and 3.4 times higher in South Asian women than in European women (12.6% compared to 3.7%) [1].

The Distribution of Diabetes in the Elderly by Socio-Economic Status

The relationship of low socio-economic status (SES) with several major risk factors associated with the development of type 2 diabetes, including obesity, physical inactivity and smoking is established. The role of SES in the development of diabetes has been explored and there is a reported inverse relationship between measures of SES and diabetes [22]. Those in the most deprived fifth of society are 2.5 times more likely to develop diabetes than those in the most affluent fifth [21]. A community-based study that looked at the relationship between SES and diabetes prevalence across different age-groups found that a marked difference in diabetes prevalence by SES was apparent in the middle-aged, and especially those aged 40–49 years. In this age-group diabetes prevalence in those in the highest (most deprived) quintile was almost double that of those in the lowest quintile, using a ward based deprivation score derived from census data on factors associated with deprivation, including unemployment, no-car households, overcrowded households and rented accommodation [23]. In the elderly the relationship of the deprivation score with diabetes prevalence was less apparent. This could be due to the higher mortality that exists in people with diabetes in more socially deprived groups [24]. In the MRC trial of assessment and management of older people in the community in individuals aged 75 years and older those in the most deprived quintile of Carstairs deprivation index had 1.3 times the risk of diabetes compared to those in the least deprived quintile [2]. In this study the relationship between SES and diabetes was not linear. Those in the third and fourth quintiles in terms of deprivation were at the highest risk of diabetes (odds ratios of 1.5 and 1.6 respectively). A plausible explanation for the weaker relationship between SES and diabetes in the elderly is that premature death from all causes is more common among those of lower SES [25].

Association of Diabetes with Morbidity in the Elderly

Data on morbidity associated with diabetes in the elderly are sparse. This may in part reflect a view that diabetes in the elderly is 'mild' diabetes and that the associated health consequences are less severe than in younger people. This is a view that has been challenged [1, 17]. The data that do exist suggest that diabetes in the elderly is associated with a similar or greater amount of morbidity as in younger populations [1]. In the MRC trial of individuals aged 75 years and older after adjustment for age, sex and smoking, those with diabetes had a higher prevalence of angina (1.3 times higher), history of myocardial infarction (1.5 times higher) and history of a cerebrovascular event (two-fold higher) than those without diabetes. Those with diabetes also had 1.6 times more visual impairment and 1.7 times more foot ulceration than those without [2]. In a Swedish cohort study of almost 600 men followed up over 10 years to the age of 67 years the incidence of coronary heart disease was over 30% in those with known diabetes, compared to 9% in those without diabetes [26]. In a population based case control study conducted in Wales and involving 403 cases (with diabetes) and 403 matched controls with a median age of 75 years those with diabetes were found to have considerably worse health than those without [27]. Those with diabetes had more vascular disease, and also worse mobility than those without. Overall those with diabetes had a mean of 2.5 co-morbidities compared to a mean of 1.9 in the control subjects [27]. National data from the United States also show a considerable excess of morbidity in elderly individuals with diabetes compared to those without. During 10 years of follow up, individuals aged 65–95 years at entry into the study who had diabetes were at excess risk of lower limb morbidity than those without. This was particularly marked for more severe conditions requiring surgery. For example, gangrene was diagnosed in 19% of those with diabetes, but in only 1% of those without diabetes. Cardiovascular disease was also significantly more common in those with diabetes compared to those without (prevalence of 70% compared to 40% respectively) [28].

Compared to elderly individuals without diabetes those with diabetes suffer excess morbidity. Elderly individuals with diabetes are at risk of developing a range of macrovascular and microvascular complications as well as functional impairment, similar to the diabetes-related morbidities experienced by younger people with the condition. In terms of the management of diabetes complications the elderly represent a special group in that lifestyle interventions related to physical activity and dietary change may be more difficult in this group and in addition cognitive complications may make adherence to a medication regimen problematic.

Association of Diabetes with Mortality in the Elderly

Given the excess morbidity associated with diabetes in the elderly it seems likely that elderly individuals with diabetes will suffer excess mortality risk. Figure 1.4 shows the excess mortality associated with diabetes reported from the

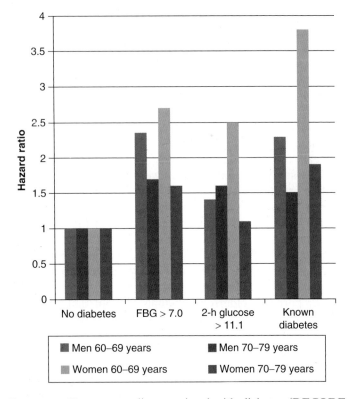

FIGURE 1.4 Excess mortality associated with diabetes (DECODE study data; adapted from [28])

DECODE study, a collaborative analysis of data from population-based studies across Europe [29]. The data show the age adjusted hazard ratio of mortality for men and women in two age-groups; 60–69 years and 70–79 years. Subjects were split into those with no diabetes, those with previously diagnosed diabetes and those found to have diabetes at screening, either on the basis of a fasting or 2-h post glucose challenge blood glucose, according to Word Health Organisation criteria [30]. Compared to the reference group (no diabetes), those with known diabetes have between 1.5 and 3.8 times the risk of mortality and those with diabetes diagnosed on the basis of fasting or post-challenge glucose up to 2.7 times the risk of mortality. Similar data reporting an excess mortality risk for elderly individuals with diabetes exist from other studies. A study of individuals aged 65 years and older living in Melton Mowbray reported that those with diabetes were 4.5 times more likely to die than those with no evidence of diabetes over 4.5 years of follow-up [9]. A community based study which identified all individuals with diabetes and followed them up over 11 years identified an SMR of 159 for those aged 65–74 years and 126 for those aged 75 years and older for all causes of death, based on England and Wales population data [31]. Data from a national longitudinal study in the United States showed that those aged 65 years and older with diabetes had excess mortality of 9.2% compared with those with no diabetes over 11 years of follow-up [28].

There is some evidence that an excess of death from cardiovascular disease occurs in elderly individuals with diabetes. Data from the Finnish cohorts of the Seven Countries Study show that in men aged 65 years and older with diabetes the relative risk of death is more than double that of men with normal glucose tolerance and that men in the 65–74 year age group had an increased risk of death from cardiovascular disease [32].

The increased risk of mortality and morbidity apparent in elderly individuals with diabetes necessitates an appropriate approach to their identification and management. The need for such an approach is particularly pertinent given that the elderly, if they are considered to be those at or above the age of 60 years, represent half of the total diabetic population of the UK [3].

Screening for and Diagnosis of Diabetes in the Elderly

Clearly it is important to identify elderly individuals who have undiagnosed diabetes who will benefit from the provision of effective medical care to minimise the serious potential health consequences of diabetes. Debate continues about population screening for diabetes and its benefits [33, 34]. Surprisingly, despite the fact that half of all people with diabetes in the UK are aged over 60 years, little is known about the potential value of screening for diabetes in this age group. It has been suggested that a benign age-related deterioration in glucose metabolism that is asymptomatic and unrelated to excess morbidity and mortality might be revealed by screening [26], raising questions about the value of screening for diabetes in elderly populations. However the evidence presented above demonstrates a substantial excess of both morbidity and mortality in elderly people with diabetes that could be reduced by earlier detection and treatment. Further studies are required to provide evidence of an appropriate level of dysglycaemia at which intervention is appropriate to reduce diabetes related morbidity and mortality in the elderly.

Agreement on an appropriate diagnostic test must also be reached. The American Diabetes Association previously recommended that fasting glucose be used for the diagnosis of diabetes and more recently that HbA_{1c} testing be used for both diagnosis and monitoring [35]. The World Health Organisation continues to recommend the use of the OGTT. The implications of using either HbA_{1c} or fasting glucose diagnostically in terms of their utility to reduce diabetes related complications in the elderly remain unclear. Elderly individuals can have lower fasting glucose values but meet post prandial criteria for the diagnosis of diabetes [36]. The use of post prandial glucose increases the number of cases of diabetes identified in the elderly compared to the use of fasting blood glucose alone [16]. This may be attributable to a reduction in insulin release in response to a glucose load. In addition in post-menopausal women the relationship between impaired fasting glucose and the development of diabetes and cardiovascular risk is less clear than in younger populations [37]. This raises the possibility that fasting glucose is less predictive of risk of morbidity and mortality in older populations and that the OGTT remains the most reliable method for identifying diabetes in the elderly [38].

Summary

The population of the UK is ageing such that it is anticipated that within 20 years approximately a quarter of the population will be aged 65 years and older. It is estimated that around 14% of men and 10% of women in this age group currently have diagnosed diabetes. As the elderly population increases the number of people living with diabetes will increase dramatically. Diabetes is more common in certain ethnic minority groups and as these ethnic groups increase in size over the next decades there will be an increasing impact on the total diabetes burden.

Elderly individuals with diabetes suffer the same health consequences and excess mortality faced by younger people with diabetes. Effective strategies to appropriately identify those who stand to benefit from early detection and treatment are needed.

References

1. Simmons D, Williams DR. Diabetes in the elderly: an under-diagnosed condition. Diabet Med. 1993;10:264–6.
2. Hewitt J, Smeeth L, Bulpitt CJ, Fletcher AE. The prevalence of Type 2 diabetes and its associated health problems in a community-dwelling elderly population. Diabet Med. 2009;26:370–6.
3. APHO. APHO Diabetes Prevalence Model: Key findings for England: YHPHO2010 June 2010.
4. Wild S, Roglic G, Green A, Sicree R, King H. Global prevalence of diabetes. Estimates for the year 2000 and projections for 2030. Diabetes Care. 2004;27:1047–53.
5. Office for National Statistics. Ageing. Fastest increase in the oldest old. 2010 [cited 2011 14 April]; Available from: http://www.statistics.gov.uk/cci/nugget.asp?ID=949.
6. Office for National Statistics. National Population Projections. 2009 [cited 2011 14 April]; Available from: http://www.statistics.gov.uk/STATBASE/Product.asp?vlnk=8519.
7. Rees P. Ethnic Population Projections: Review and Illustration of Issues. 2007 [cited 2011 14 April]; Available from: http://www.ccsr.ac.uk/events/segint/workshops/documents/PhilReesEthnicPopulationProjectionsCCSRworkshop.pdf.

8. Mather HM, Keen H. The Southall Diabetes Survey: prevalence of known diabetes in Asians and Europeans. BMJ. 1985;291:1081–4.

9. Croxson SC, Jagger C. Diabetes and cognitive impairment: a community-based study of elderly subjects. Age Ageing. 1995;24:421–4.

10. Hayes L, Hawthorne G, Unwin N. Undiagnosed diabetes in the over-60s: performance of the APHO diabetes prevalence model in a general practice. Diabetic Medicine. 2011 (in press).

11. Thomas MC, Hardoon SL, Papacosta AO, Morris RW, Wannamethee SG, Sloggett A, et al. Evidence of an accelerating increase in prevalence of diagnosed Type 2 diabetes in British men, 1978–2005. Diabet Med. 2009;26:766–72.

12. Zimmet P, Alberti KG, Shaw J. Global and societal implications of the diabetes epidemic. Nature. 2001;414:782–7.

13. Holman NF, N.G. Goyder, E., Wild SH. The Association of Public Health Observatories (APHO) Diabetes Prevalence Model: estimates of total diabetes prevalence for England, 2010–2030. Diabet Med 2011;Accepted Article; doi: 10.1111/j.1464-5491.2010.03216.x.

14. Collerton J, Davies K, Jagger C, Kingston A, Bond J, Eccles MP, et al. Health and disease in 85 year olds: baseline findings from the Newcastle 85+ cohort study. BMJ. 2009;339:b4904.

15. The Information Centre. National Diabetes Audit 2004/5. Leeds: The Information Centre 2006.

16. Aspray TJ, Nesbit K, Cassidy TP, Farrow E, Hawthorne G. Diabetes in British nursing and residential homes: a pragmatic screening study. Diabetes Care. 2006;29:707–8.

17. Sinclair AJ, Gadsby R, Penfold S, Croxson SC, Bayer AJ. Prevalence of diabetes in care home residents. Diabetes Care. 2001;24:1066–8.

18. Ruwaard D, Gijsen R, Bartelds AI, Hirasing RA, Verkleij H, Kromhout D. Is the incidence of diabetes increasing in all age-groups in The Netherlands? Results of the second study in the Dutch Sentinel Practice Network. Diabetes Care. 1996;19:214–8.

19. Rockwood K, Awalt E, MacKnight C, McDowell I. Incidence and outcomes of diabetes mellitus in elderly people: report from the Canadian Study of Health and Aging. CMAJ. 2000;162:769–72.

20. Vanderpump MP, Tunbridge WM, French JM, Appleton D, Bates D, Rodgers H, et al. The incidence of diabetes mellitus in an English community: a 20-year follow-up of the Whickham Survey. Diabet Med. 1996;13:741–7.

21. Health Survey for England. Health Survey for England 2004: The Health of Minority Ethnic Groups. London: Department of Health 2004 6 March 2007.

22. Kumari M, Head J, Marmot M. Prospective study of social and other risk factors for incidence of type 2 diabetes in the Whitehall II study. Arch Intern Med. 2004 27;164:1873–80.

23. Connolly V, Unwin N, Sherriff P, Bilous R, Kelly W. Diabetes prevalence and socioeconomic status: a population based study showing increased prevalence of type 2 diabetes mellitus in deprived areas. J Epidemiol Community Health. 2000;54:173–7.

24. Connolly V, Kelly W. Risk factors for diabetes in men. Risk factors are closely linked with socioeconomic status. BMJ. 1995;311:188.
25. Chaturvedi N, Jarrett J, Shipley MJ, Fuller JH. Socioeconomic gradient in morbidity and mortality in people with diabetes: cohort study findings from the Whitehall Study and the WHO Multinational Study of Vascular Disease in Diabetes. BMJ. 1998;316:100–5.
26. Welin L, Eriksson H, Larsson B, Ohlson LO, Svardsudd K, Tibblin G. Hyperinsulinaemia is not a major coronary risk factor in elderly men. The study of men born in 1913. Diabetologia. 1992;35:766–70.
27. Sinclair AJ, Conroy SP, Bayer AJ. Impact of diabetes on physical function in older people. Diabetes Care. 2008;31:233–5.
28. Bethel MA, Sloan FA, Belsky D, Feinglos MN. Longitudinal incidence and prevalence of adverse outcomes of diabetes mellitus in elderly patients. Arch Intern Med. 2007;167:921–7.
29. DECODE Study Group. Consequences of the new diagnostic criteria for diabetes in older men and women. DECODE Study (Diabetes Epidemiology: Collaborative Analysis of Diagnostic Criteria in Europe). Diabetes Care. 1999;22:1667–71.
30. World Health Organization and International Diabetes Federation. Definition, diagnosis and classification of diabetes mellitus and its complications. Geneva: WHO1999.
31. Walters DP, Gatling W, Houston AC, Mullee MA, Julious SA, Hill RD. Mortality in diabetic subjects: an eleven-year follow-up of a community-based population. Diabet Med. 1994;11:968–73.
32. Stengard JH, Tuomilehto J, Pekkanen J, Kivinen P, Kaarsalo E, Nissinen A, et al. Diabetes mellitus, impaired glucose tolerance and mortality among elderly men: the Finnish cohorts of the Seven Countries Study. Diabetologia. 1992;35:760–5.
33. Wareham NJ, Griffin SJ. Should we screen for type 2 diabetes? Evaluation against National Screening Committee criteria. BMJ. 2001;322:986–8.
34. Goyder EC. Screening for and prevention of type 2 diabetes. BMJ. 2008;336:1140–1.
35. American Diabetes Association. Diagnosis and Classification of Diabetes Mellitus. Diabetes Care. 2010;33(Suppl 1):S62–S9.
36. Wahl PW, Savage PJ, Psaty BM, Orchard TJ, Robbins JA, Tracy RP. Diabetes in older adults: comparison of 1997 American Diabetes Association classification of diabetes mellitus with 1985 WHO classification. Lancet. 1998;352:1012–5.
37. Kanaya AM, Herrington D, Vittinghoff E, Lin F, Bittner V, Cauley JA, et al. Impaired fasting glucose and cardiovascular outcomes in postmenopausal women with coronary artery disease. Summary for patients in Ann Intern Med. 2005;142:813–820
38. DECODE Study Group. Will new diagnostic criteria for diabetes mellitus change phenotype of patients with diabetes? Reanalysis of European epidemiological data. DECODE Study Group on behalf of the European Diabetes Epidemiology Study Group. BMJ. 1998; 317:371–5.

Chapter 2
Type 2 Diabetes and Dementia

Mark W.J. Strachan

Introduction

Dementia is a devastating illness. Not only does it rob an individual of his or her memory, but it also takes away that individual's independence and can have dramatic effects on family and friends. Eighteen percent of deaths in men and 23% of deaths in women aged 85–89 years are directly attributable to dementia. Over the age of 65 years, the prevalence of dementia doubles every 5 years so that, for example, 5.9% of people aged 75–79 years and 12.2% of people aged 80–84 years are affected. Current estimates suggest that 700,000 people in the United Kingdom (1.1% of the population) have dementia and that this figure will rise to over 1.7 million by 2051 (Fig. 2.1) [1]. Among people aged over 60, dementia contributes 11.2% of all years lived with disability, more than stroke (9.5%), musculoskeletal disorders (8.9%), cardiovascular disease (5.0%) and cancer (2.4%). The proportion of individuals with dementia living in care homes rises with age – 26.% of those aged 65–74 years compared with 60.8% of those aged 90 years or older. Leaving aside the human element, in financial terms, dementia currently costs the UK economy a staggering £17 billion per annum – that is

M.W.J. Strachan
Metabolic Unit, Western General Hospital,
Crewe Road, Edinburgh, EH4 2XU, UK

G. Hawthorne (ed.), *Diabetes Care for the Older Patient*,
DOI 10.1007/978-0-85729-461-6_2,
© Springer-Verlag London Limited 2012

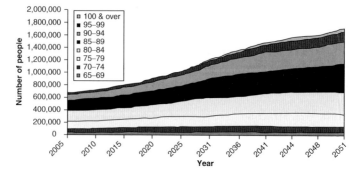

FIGURE 2.1 Projected increases in the number of people in the UK with dementia, by age group (2005–2051) (Reproduced from the 'Dementia UK Full Report, 2007' [1], with permission from the Alzheimer's Society)

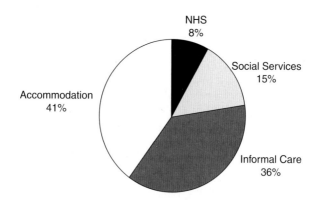

FIGURE 2.2 The distribution of dementia service costs (Reproduced from the 'Dementia UK Full Report, 2007' [1], with permission from the Alzheimer's Society)

on average £25,000 per person with dementia [1]. These figures include loss of income (and taxes paid to the Exchequer) from carers and costs for accommodation, NHS and social services (Fig. 2.2). Thus, dementia represents an enormous issue for our society now, but this will increase dramatically in the years to come as the numbers of affected individuals relentlessly rises.

Causes of Dementia

The 'brain damage' that leads to dementia may be the end-result of many different and unrelated disease processes and is often preceded by a lower level of cognitive dysfunction, which is sometimes termed 'Mild Cognitive Impairment' (MCI) [2]. The commonest cause of dementia is Alzheimer's disease (AD), which accounts for about 60% of cases. Vascular dementia (VaD) and mixed forms of dementia account for about 30% and the remainder are made up of rarer forms, such as dementia with Lewy bodies and fronto-temporal dementia (neither of which are discussed further in this chapter).

In AD, characteristic neuroanatomical abnormalities are observed in the form of senile plaques and neurofibrillary tangles of hyperphosphorylated tau protein. The senile plaques contain β-amyloid protein and it is thought that deposition of this protein is the initial mechanism that results in the deterioration of neuronal synapse function, composition, and structure [3]. Early-onset AD (occurring before the age of 60 years) is rare and is caused by fully penetrant mutations in three autosomal dominant genes: Aβ-precursor protein, presenilin 1 and presenilin 2 [4]. However, most cases of AD are late-onset and are not associated with a strong family history. It is likely that genetic predisposition to late-onset AD is mediated by highly prevalent genetic variants of low penetrance in a number of different genes, in the same way that multiple different genetic variants are thought to predispose to Type 2 diabetes. The most established of these is the Apolipoprotein E (APOE) gene. Inheritance of one copy of the APOE ε4 allele increases risk of AD by a factor of 3, whereas homozygosity is associated with a 12-fold increase in risk [5]. APOE is, however, neither sufficient nor necessary for the development of AD. The advent of high-density genome-wide association studies has resulted in the identification of a whole array of novel genetic risk alleles and variants for dementia [4].

VaD is a heterogeneous term for many different processes that result in dementia because of cerebral infarction, hypoperfusion or haemorrhage [6]. Large vessel vascular dementia is usually embolic in nature and the cognitive impairment may result from cerebral damage through numerous infarcts, which are widely distributed throughout the brain (multi-infarct dementia) or a single infarct in a critical area of the brain (strategic-infarct dementia). The most common form though is a consequence of cerebral small vessel disease (subcortical ischaemic vascular dementia) and is associated with the presence of lacunar infarcts and white matter lesions [6, 7].

Differentiating between AD and VaD can be difficult in a clinical setting. Some diagnostic tips are shown at the end of the chapter. Typically a history of sudden-onset dementia or a step-wise deterioration in cognitive function favours VaD, whereas in AD the decline is more gradual and memory loss may predominate over impairment in other cognitive domains. However, there is a substantial clinical overlap between these two syndromes. MRI studies have demonstrated that 'silent' vascular lesions are extremely common in older people [6] and neuropathological investigations have shown that most individuals with dementia actually have a mixed AD and VaD pattern [8].

Risk Factors for Dementia

In recent years, our understanding of the risk factors for dementia has increased significantly, particularly through well-constructed population-based studies [9]. As has already been alluded to, age is the most important risk factor for dementia and genetic predisposition is also important. Higher levels of education may be protective as may be a 'Mediterranean' diet, moderate alcohol consumption, regular exercise and caffeine. Epidemiological studies have also suggested a protective effect of non-steroidal anti-inflammatory drugs and hormone-replacement therapy in post-menopausal women. Head injury doubles the risk of AD, while an increased risk of both AD and VaD is associated with cardiovascular disease and its classic risk factors, e.g., obesity, hypertension, dyslipidaemia, elevated plasma homocysteine and, of primary relevance to this article, diabetes.

In a 7 year, prospective study of 1,433 people in France aged over 65 years [9], diabetes was associated with a hazard ratio of 1.85 (95% confidence interval 1.34–2.56) for incident MCI or dementia and it was calculated that diabetes accounted for 4.9% of the overall risk (the adjusted population attributable fraction (PAF)). In this study, the other key risk factors for MCI and dementia identified were low crystallised intelligence (PAF 18.1%), depression (PAF 10.3%), consumption of fruit and vegetables less than twice per day (PAF 6.5%) and presence of an APOE 4 ε4 allele (PAF 7.1%).

Thus the magnitude of the effect of diabetes on risk of dementia is comparable to that of its main established genetic risk factor. Although the effect size is not enormous, diabetes represents a modifiable risk factor (unlike genetic risk factors) and because diabetes is so prevalent in the general population, any intervention that reduced the number of people developing diabetes would have a high impact on the incidence of MCI and dementia and would be cost effective. The relationship between dementia, depression and diabetes will be discussed later in this chapter. The authors of this study concluded that interventions to increase crystallised intelligence and fruit and vegetable consumption would be difficult to formulate at a population level and that 'in the continued absence of an effective treatment for the dementias, public health programmes should aim above all at prevention of diabetes [9]...'

Healthcare professionals who are contending with the dramatic increase in numbers of people with Type 2 diabetes might smile at the apparent naivety of the above statement. Indeed, the number of people with diabetes over the age of 65 years in the developed world is expected to rise from 25 to 48 million over the next 30 years [10]. Thus, the nightmare scenario is that if these estimates come to pass, then the predictions for the future numbers of people with dementia might turn out to be substantially underestimated. In the absence of a clearly identified public health diabetes prevention strategy, we need to understand better the mechanisms underpinning the relationship between diabetes and dementia. Only by doing so can we hope to identify appropriate preventative and therapeutic strategies.

Why is Type 2 Diabetes only now being recognised as a Risk factor for Dementia?

Early literature suggested that diabetes was actually *less* common in people with dementia, but this was almost certainly a manifestation of survival bias, because people with diabetes were dying prematurely before they had lived long enough to develop dementia. People are now living to increasingly advanced ages with diabetes because of better prevention and treatment of the classic micro- and macrovascular complications. This means that people have diabetes for increasingly longer durations and so hitherto unrecognised complications of diabetes, such as dementia, may start to appear.

The potential for 'novel' complications of diabetes to declare themselves will be more likely if they are less responsive to current treatment algorithms than 'conventional' complications. In that regard, cognitive impairment and dementia appear to be stubbornly resistant to the effects of therapies targeting cardiovascular risk factors, which is surprising given that vascular mechanisms undoubtedly play a role in their genesis. Thus, statin therapy given late in life to individuals at risk of vascular disease has no effect in preventing dementia [11]. Randomised trials have shown no evidence that aspirin reduces cognitive decline in either healthy women aged over 65 years [12] or middle aged to elderly adults with asymptomatic atherosclerosis [13]. Moreover, a Cochrane review found no convincing evidence that antihypertensive drugs prevented the development of dementia in hypertensive patients without prior cerebrovascular disease [14]. One chink of light in favour of antihypertensive drugs came from the PROGRESS trial, where therapy with perindopril and indapamide was associated with a lower risk of dementia (34%) and cognitive decline (45%) in people with cerebrovascular disease; this effect was mediated by reducing the incidence of recurrent stroke [15]. It should be stressed though that the disappointing trial data relate to therapies being given to older people. It is entirely conceivable that very prolonged statin, anti-platelet and anti-hypertensive therapy (i.e. therapies initiated in middle age) could have long-term benefits on the incidence of cognitive impairment and dementia, but this remains untested in randomized trials.

There are other reasons why dementia may not have been recognised hitherto as a complication of diabetes. Mild levels of cognitive impairment may not be evident when a person is reviewed in the context of a routine diabetes check-up, particularly when an individual has been reviewed by many different doctors over the years. Moreover, routine screening for cognitive impairment is not performed at a diabetes review in most centres. Finally, as individuals become increasingly frail and cognitively impaired, they may no longer be able to attend for routine diabetes review. It is, therefore, only with the advent of large-scale community-based epidemiological studies, in which sophisticated cognitive testing has been performed, that the relationship between diabetes, cognitive impairment and dementia has become apparent.

Why is dementia more common in People with Type 2 Diabetes?

Type 2 diabetes is a remarkably complex metabolic disorder, so it is inevitable that the aetiology of cognitive impairment and dementia associated with diabetes will be multifactorial in nature [16–18]. Some of the potential risk factors are demonstrated in Fig. 2.3. It is beyond the scope of this chapter to consider all of these in detail, so the remainder of this chapter will focus on genetic factors, hyperglycaemia, cerebral microvascular disease, hypoglycaemia and depression.

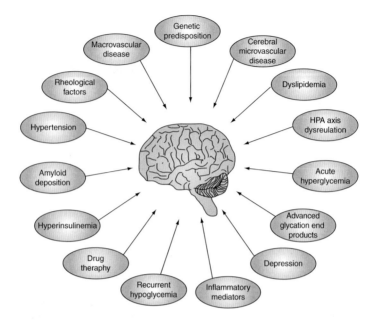

FIGURE 2.3 Risk factors for cognitive impairment and dementia in Type 2 diabetes (Reproduced from Strachan et al. Nature Reviews Endocrinology 2011 [17], with permission from the Nature Publishing Group)

Genetic Factors

Our genes cannot be modified, but as has already been described they can significantly influence our risk of developing dementia. In a study of 826 community-dwelling individuals, cognitive function was found to be poorer in people with diabetes than in those individuals who did not have diabetes [19]. Intriguingly, this negative association between diabetes and cognition was significantly *greater* in those individuals who carried one or more APOE ε4 alleles (Fig. 2.4), i.e. genetic factors further moderated the association between diabetes and cognitive impairment.

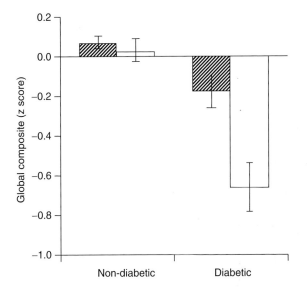

FIGURE 2.4 Effects of Apolipoprotein E genotype on cognition in people with and without diabetes The *shaded bars* represent individuals who are negative for Apolipoprotein E ε4 genotype, while the *open bars* are for individuals who have at least one Apolipoprotein E ε4 allele. The y-axis shows a global composite cognitive function z-score, which has a mean of 0 and a standard deviation of ±1. Negative scores represent poorer cognition. Individuals with diabetes who were Apolipoprotein E ε4 positive had the poorest cognitive function (Reproduced from Dore et al. 2009 [19], with permission from Springer Verlag)

Hyperglycaemia

Some people with diabetes report that they do not feel well when their blood glucose concentrations are elevated and, aside from the classic osmotic symptoms, a commonly reported symptom is poor concentration. In an experimental clamp study in people with Type 2 diabetes, this observation was supported, such that when plasma glucose was raised from normoglycaemia to 16.5 mmol/l decrements in working memory and attention were observed, along with reduced levels of happiness and energy, and increased levels of tension [20]. The mechanism of this very acute effect of hyperglycaemia is not known, but could conceivably be mediated by alterations in regional cerebral blood flow and/or osmotic changes in cerebral neurones.

Data from two relatively short-term randomised controlled trials suggest that improvements in glycaemic control may affect cognitive function. In one study, 141 adults with Type 2 diabetes treated with metfomin were randomised to receive additional therapy with glibenclamide or rosiglitazone over 26 weeks. Working memory improved in both arms of the study, with no change observed in tests of mental efficiency or learning ability. Those subjects with the greatest improvement in glycaemic control had the greatest improvement in working memory [21]. In another study, 156 adults with treatment-naive Type 2 diabetes were randomised to receive either repaglinide or glibenclamide [22]. Over 1 year of follow up, executive and attention function declined in the glibenclamide group, but not the repaglinide group, and this decline was abolished statistically after adjustment for postprandial hyperglycaemia.

Cognitive function was included as an end-point in two much larger randomised trials, ADVANCE and ACCORD, which also had a more prolonged period of follow-up than those above. Cognition was, though, only one of many end-points and so necessarily the detail of the cognitive assessment was reduced. In the ADVANCE trial, cognition was assessed by means of the Mini Mental State Examination (MMSE) alone [23]. Subjects were randomised to conventional glycaemic control or to intensive glucose control based on modified-release GLICLAZIDE, aiming for a target HbA1c of ≤6.5% [48 mmol/mol]. There was also an intensive blood pressure control part of the trial, based around perindopril-indapamide or placebo. Neither the intensive glucose nor the intensive blood pressure intervention modified the risk of cognitive decline or dementia. The participants, at baseline, had much better glycaemic control than those in the smaller studies above and it may well be that the benefits of improvements in glycaemia were only manifest when glucose was reduced from relatively high levels. Moreover, the MMSE is only a very crude marker of cognitive impairment may not have been sufficiently sensitive to detect any mild to moderate changes in cognitive function. Intensive glycaemic control was also, predictably, associated with an increased risk of hypoglycaemia and it is also conceivable that any beneficial effects of improved glycaemia on cognition may have been counterbalanced by increased hypoglycaemia (see below).

Cognitive function was assessed in a more detailed fashion in the ACCORD study and in the baseline assessment there was an association between higher HbA1c and poorer cognition [24]. The prospective cognitive data from this trial are yet to be published, though may be of more limited value following the early termination of the glucose-lowering arm of this study [25].

Cerebral Small Vessel Disease

Microvascular disease is one of the pathognomonic complications of diabetes and it is probable that this occurs in the brain as well as in peripheral organs. Cerebral small vessel disease is implicated in the pathogenesis of lacunar stroke and it is not an enormous leap of faith to speculate that it might also be associated with cognitive impairment and dementia. Cerebral microvascular disease is likely to be caused by both chronic hyperglycaemia and hypertension, but is something that is not easy to assess directly *in vivo*. However, the small vessels of the retina share similar embryological origin, size, structure and physiological characteristic to the small vessels of the brain (including a blood-retinal barrier which is analogous to the blood-brain barrier) [26, 27]. Thus, the vessels of the retina have the potential to provide a surrogate measure of the state of the cerebral microvasculature. Several large epidemiological studies have linked retinal microvascular abnormalities with cognitive impairment in the general population [28–30].

In the Edinburgh Type 2 Diabetes Study (ET2DS), a population-based epidemiological study of risk factors for

cognitive impairment in Type 2 diabetes, a significant association in men was found between the degree of diabetic retinopathy and cognitive function, such that poorer cognition was
linked with higher levels of retinopathy [31]. This would
clearly support the hypothesis that cerebral microvascular
disease causes cognitive impairment. However, another interpretation of these data is that people with poorer cognition
were less able to achieve strict glycaemic control and that
predisposed them to develop diabetic retinopathy (reverse
causality). A third possible explanation is that the relationship between retinopathy and cognition was confounded by
another factor that predisposed to both of these factors – for
example, people with diabetic retinopathy tended to have
longer duration of diabetes and were more likely to have
hypertension. Longitudinal data are clearly needed to con-
firm or refute each of these three interpretations, although
the ET2DS investigators favoured the first explanation as the
relationship between retinopathy and cognition remained
even after adjustment for potential confounding factors and
pre-morbid (or best-ever) intelligence.

Hypoglycaemia

A number of cross-sectional studies in the 1990s reported
that, in people with Type 1 diabetes, recurrent exposure to
severe hypoglycaemia was associated with modest cognitive decrements [32]. However, in the 18-year follow up of
the DCCT cohort, no relationship was observed between
the frequency of severe hypoglycaemia and cognitive function [33]. Life-time exposure to severe hypoglycaemia is
much lower in people with Type 2 diabetes than in Type 1
diabetes, and if no long-term effect has been seen on cognitive function in people with Type 1 diabetes, it would seem
improbable that severe hypoglycaemia could cause cognitive
decline in people with Type 2 diabetes. However, recent data
from the United States have challenged this presumption.
In a study of 16,667 adults with Type 2 diabetes who were
members of a North Californian diabetes register [34], a

dose–response relationship was observed between the frequency of severe hypoglycaemia and the risk of developing dementia (Table 2.1). This effect held true after adjustment for HbA1c and co-morbidities such as cardiovascular disease and end-stage renal disease. There were significant limitations to this study – data were collected retrospectively from electronic records, without any direct assessment of the subjects, and adjustment for potential confounding factors was relatively limited. There is also the possibility of reverse causality, i.e., people with cognitive impairment might be more prone to have episodes of severe hypoglycaemia, because of reduced self-caring behaviours. Indeed, in the ADVANCE study, participants with a MMSE score of ≤23 were two-fold more likely to experience an episode of severe hypoglycaemia during the period of follow-up, even after adjustment for age, sex, treatment allocation and educational status [23]. Similarly in the Fremantle Diabetes Study, dementia was associated with a three-fold increased risk of hypoglycaemia requiring health service use over a mean 3.7 years of follow-up [35]. However, the authors of the North Californian study did attempt to address the issue of reverse causality by performing 'lag' analyses, and in these the relationship between severe hypoglycaemia and incident dementia remained [34].

As stated previously, it does seem implausible at first glance that severe hypoglycaemia might cause cognitive decrements in

TABLE 2.1 Relationship between the risk of developing dementia and the frequency of severe hypoglycaemia

Episodes of hypoglycaemia	HR	95% CI
0	1	
1	1.26	1.10–1.49
2	1.80	1.37–1.26
3 or more	1.94	1.42–2.64

Data from Whitmer et al. [34]. Reproduced from Strachan, *Diabetic Medicine* [18] with permission from Wiley
HR – adjusted hazard ratios for risk of developing dementia, *CI* confidence intervals

people with Type 2 diabetes, but not in people with Type 1 diabetes. However, it must be remembered that the DCCT cohort were young at recruitment and had little in the way of co-morbidities [33]. It is quite conceivable that the older brain of an individual with Type 2 diabetes, which has already been exposed to a lifetime of toxic insults and which has to contend with all the other co-morbidities associated with Type 2 diabetes, could be especially vulnerable to the effects of severe hypoglycaemia.

Depression

The association between dementia and depression is well recognised. It is common in the general population and is relatively easy to treat. Symptoms of depression may precede a clinical diagnosis of dementia, but what is not clear is whether dementia is a risk factor for dementia or whether it is simply an early feature of dementia itself [9]. Depression is also more common in people with Type 2 diabetes [36] and it is similarly not clear whether this association is related to a specific biological mechanism or simply because depression is more common in people who have chronic medical disorders. In the Edinburgh Type 2 Diabetes Study, symptoms of depression (assessed using the Hospital Anxiety and Depression Scale) were negatively associated with cognitive function ($r = -0.2$) and were independently associated with symptoms of anxiety, increasing central obesity, the presence of ischaemic heart disease and the need for insulin therapy [37].

There is substantial evidence that the hypothalamic-pituitary-adrenal (HPA) axis is dysregulated in people with depression [38]. It is also well established that people with Type 2 diabetes have activation of the HPA axis, with elevated basal plasma cortisol levels [39, 40], higher salivary cortisol levels [41], elevated ACTH levels [42], increased plasma cortisol levels following overnight dexamethasone [43, 44] and impaired habituation of cortisol levels to repeated stress [45]. Few studies have specifically examined the relationship between diabetes, depression and the HPA axis, but in one study [46], which included subjects both with and without diabetes, an association was observed between higher plasma cortisol levels, more depressive symptoms and higher glucose concentrations. This effect was stronger in African Americans who are known to have a high incidence of both diabetes and depression.

It is relatively easy to screen for depression at a population level and whether or not it represents a dementia prodrome and whether or not it is a specific feature of diabetes, treatment of depression should diminish the rate of functional loss associated with dementia.

Is There Sufficient Evidence to Warrant Screening for Cognitive Impairment and Dementia in People with Diabetes?

As is well known, screening for a given disorder should only be undertaken if there is a good screening test and if detection will lead to an intervention that will improve outcomes for the individual. While there are screening tests available for cognitive impairment, such as the MMSE and the Abbreviated Mental Test, they are relatively crude and are difficult to assess as one-off measures. Currently licensed therapies for dementia have, at best, a moderate impact on cognitive function and do not modify the natural history of cognitive decline. Thus, it is difficult to justify routine screening for dementia at present, although clinicians should maintain a high index of suspicion. As has already been discussed, screening for depression is feasible and there are effective treatments; therefore, screening is routinely undertaken in people with diabetes in many primary and secondary care services.

Conclusions

It is now well-established that Type 2 diabetes is an important risk factor dementia, indeed epidemiological data suggest that prevention of diabetes would have a significant public health benefit in terms of reducing incident MCI and dementia. At present though, strategies to prevent diabetes are failing and the incidence of both diabetes and dementia is set to rise dramatically in the coming decades. We need to understand better why Type 2 diabetes is associated with dementia, because only by understanding the mechanisms involved can the rational design of future preventative and therapeutic strategies be informed. Some data suggest that improving glycaemic control may be beneficial in enhancing cognitive function, but hypoglycaemia may be particularly damaging to the vulnerable brains of older people with Type 2 diabetes. Cerebral small vessel disease has also been implicated, while low mood may either promote the development of dementia or be an early symptom of cognitive impairment.

Practical Points

Criteria to help make a diagnosis of dementia
- Decline from a previously higher level of cognitive function
- Impairment of memory and at least one other cognitive domain
- Cognitive deficits must impair activities of daily living
- Alzheimer's dementia is suggested by a continuous decline in cognitive function, with no other neurological disorder that accounts for the cognitive changes
- Vascular dementia suggested by onset of dementia within 3 months of a recognised stroke, a stepwise decline in cognitive function or fluctuating, stepwise progression of cognitive deficits.

References

1. Personal Social Services Research Unit. Dementia UK. 2007. Available at: www.alzheimers.org.uk/News_and_Campaigns/Campaigning/PDF/Dementia_UK_Full_Report.pdf, accessed 14.02.11
2. Mariani E, Monastero R and Mecocci P. Mild cognitive impairment: a systematic review. *J Alzheimers Dis* 2007; 12:23–35.

3. Zhao WQ, De Felice FG, Fernandez S et al. Amyloid beta oligomers induce impairment of neuronal insulin receptors. *FASEB J* 2008; 22: 246–260.

4. Waring SC, Rosenberg RN. Genome-wide association studies in Alzheimer disease. *Arch Neurology* 2008;65:329–334.

5. Patterson C, Feightner JW, Garcia A, Robin Hsiung G-Y, MacKnight C, Dessa Sadovnick A. Diagnosis and treatment of dementia. 1. Risk assessment and primary prevention of Alzheimer disease. *CMAJ* 2008; 178: 548–556.

6. Román GC, Erkinjuntti T, Wallin A, Pantoni L, Chui HC. Subcortical ischaemic vascular dementia. *Lancet Neurology* 2002; 1: 426–436.

7. Chui H. Subcortical ischemic vascular dementia (SIVD). *Neurology Clin* 2007; 25: 717–740.

8. Fernando MS, Ince PG for the MRC Cognitive Function and Ageing Neuropathology Study Group. Vascular pathologies and cognition in a population-based cohort of elderly people. *J Neurol Sci* 2004; 226: 13–17.

9. Ritchie K, Carrière I, Ritchie CW, Berr C, Artero S, Ancelin M-L. Designing prevention programmes to reduce incidence of dementia: prospective cohort study of modifiable risk factors. *BMJ* 2010; 341:c3885.

10. Wild S, Roglic G, Green A, Sicree R, King, H. Global prevalence of diabetes. Estimates for the year 2000 and projections for 2030. *Diabetes Care* 2004; 27: 1047–1053.

11. McGuiness B, Craig D, Bullock R and Passmore P. Statins for prevention of dementia. *Cochrane Database Syst Rev* 2009; (2): CD003160 (2009).

12. Kang JH, Cook N, Manson J, Buring JE and Grodstein F. Low dose aspirin and cognitive function in the women's health study cognitive cohort. *BMJ* 2007; **334**: 987.

13. Price JF, Stewart MC, Deary IJ, Murray GD, Sandercock P, Butcher I, Fowkes FG and AAA Trialists. Low dose aspirin and cognitive function in middle aged to elderly adults: randomised controlled trial. *BMJ* 2008; **337**: a1198.

14. McGuiness B, Todd S, Passmore P and Bullock R. Blood pressure lowering in patients without prior cerebrovascular disease for prevention of cognitive impairment and dementia. *Cochrane Database Syst Rev* 2009; (4): CD004034.

15. Tzourio C, Anderson C, Chapman N, Woodward M, Neal B, MacMahon S, Chalmers J. Effects of blood pressure lowering with perindopril and indapamide therapy on dementia and cognitive decline in patients with cerebrovascular disease. *Arch Intern Med* 2003; **163**: 1069–1075.

16. Strachan MWJ, Deary IJ, Ewing FME, Frier BM. Is type 2 (non-insulin dependent) diabetes mellitus associated with a decline in

cognitive function? A critical review of published studies. *Diabetes Care* 1997; 20: 438–445.

17. Strachan MWJ, Reynolds RM, Marioni RE, Price JF. Cognitive function, dementia and diabetes in the elderly. *Nature Reviews Endocrinology* 2011; 7: 108–114.

18. Strachan MWJ. The Brain as a target organ in Type 2 Diabetes: exploring the links with cognitive impairment and dementia. *Diabetic Medicine* 2011; 28(2): 141–7.

19. Dore GA, Elias MF, Robbins MA, Elias PK, Nagy Z. Presence of the *APOE ε4* allele modifies the relationship between type 2 diabetes and cognitive performance: the Maine–Syracuse Study. *Diabetologia* 2009; 52: 2551–2560.

20. Sommerfield AJ, Deary IJ, Frier BM. Acute hyperglycemia alters mood state and impairs cognitive performance in people with type 2 diabetes. *Diabetes Care* 2004; 27: 2335–2340.

21. Ryan CM, Fried MI, Rood JA, Cobitz AR, Waterhouse BR, Strachan MWJ. Improving metabolic control leads to better working memory in adults with Type 2 diabetes. *Diabetes Care* 2006; 29: 345–351.

22. Abbatecola AM, Rizzo MR, Barbieri M, et al. Postprandial plasma glucose excursions and cognitive functioning in aged type 2 diabetics. *Neurology* 2006; 67: 235–240.

23. de Galan BE, Zoungas S, Chalmers J, Anderson C, Dufouil C, Pillai A, Cooper M, Grobbee DE, Hackett M, Hamet P, Heller SR, Lisheng L, Macmahon S, Mancia G, Neal B, Pan CY, Patel A, Poulter N, Travert F, Woodward M; ADVANCE Collaborative Group. Cognitive function and risks of cardiovascular disease and hypoglycaemia in patients with type 2 diabetes: the Action in Diabetes and Vascular Disease: Preterax and Diamicron Modified Release Controlled Evaluation (ADVANCE) trial. *Diabetologia* 2009; **52**: 2328–2336.

24. Cukierman-Yaffe T, Gerstein HC, Williamson JD, Lazar RM, Lovato L, Miller ME, Coker LH, Murray A, Sullivan MD, Marcovina SM, Launer LJ; Action to Control Cardiovascular Risk in Diabetes-Memory in Diabetes (ACCORD-MIND) Investigators. Relationship between baseline glycemic control and cognitive function in individuals with type 2 diabetes and other cardiovascular risk factors: the action to control cardiovascular risk in diabetes-memory in diabetes (ACCORD-MIND) trial. *Diabetes Care* 2009; **32**: 221–226.

25. Action to Control Cardiovascular Risk in Diabetes Study Group. Effects of intensive glucose lowering in type 2 diabetes. *NEJM* 2008; **358**: 2545–2559.

26. Patton N, Aslam T, MacGillivray T, Pattie A, Deary IJ, Dhillon B. Retinal vascular image analysis as a potential screening tool for cerebrovascular disease : a rationale based on homology between cerebral and retinal microvasculatures. *J Anat* 2005; **206**: 319–348.

27. Kwa VI, van der Sande JJ, Stam J, Tijmes N, Vrooland JL. Retinal arterial changes correlate with cerebral small-vessel disease. *Neurology* 2002; **59**: 1536–1540.
28. Liew G, Mitchell P, Wong TY et al. Retinal microvascular signs and cognitive impairment. *J Am Geriatr Soc* 2009; 57: 1892–1896.
29. Baker ML, Marino Larsen EK, Kuller LH et al. Retinal microvascular signs, cognitive function, and dementia in older persons. *Stroke* 2007; **38**: 2041–2047.
30. Lesage SR, Mosley TH, Wong TY et al. Retinal microvascular abnormalities and cognitive decline The ARIC 14-year follow-up study. *Neurology* 2009; **73**: 862–868.
31. Ding J, Strachan MWJ, Reynolds RM et al. Diabetic retinopathy and cognitive decline in older people with type 2 diabetes: the Edinburgh Type 2 Diabetes Study. *Diabetes* 2010; 59: 2883–2889.
32. Deary IJ, Frier BM. Severe hypoglycaemia and cognitive impairment in diabetes. Link not proven. *Br Med J* 1996; **313**: 767–768.
33. Diabetes Control and Complications Trial/Epidemiology of Diabetes Interventions and Complications (DCCT/EDIC) Study Research Group. Long-term effect of diabetes and its treatment on cognitive function. *New Engl J Med* 2007; **356**: 1842–1852.
34. Whitmer RA, Karter AJ, Yaffe K, Quesenberry CP Jr, Selby JV. Hypoglycemic episodes and risk of dementia in older patients with type 2 diabetes mellitus. *JAMA* 2009; **301**; 1565–1572.
35. Bruce DG, Davis WA, Casey GP et al. Severe hypoglycaemia and cognitive impairment in older patients with diabetes: the Fremantle Diabetes Study. *Diabetologia* 2009; **52**: 1808–1815.
36. Pirraglia PA, Gupta S. The interaction of depression and diabetes: a review. *Curr Diabetes Rev* 2007; 3: 249–251.
37. Labad J, Price JF, Strachan MW, Fowkes FG, Ding J, Deary IJ, Lee AJ, Frier BM, Seckl JR, Walker BR, Reynolds RM Symptoms of depression but not anxiety are associated with central obesity and cardiovascular disease in people with type 2 diabetes: the Edinburgh Type 2 Diabetes Study. *Diabetologia* 2010; **53**: 467–471.
38. Zunszain PA, Anacker C, Cattaneo A, Carvalho LA, Pariante CM Glucocorticoids, cytokines and brain abnormalities in depression. *Prog Neuropsychopharmacol Biol Psychiatry* 2011; **35**:722–729.
39. Lee ZS, Chan JC, Yeung VT, Chow CC, Lau MS, Ko GT, Li JK, Cockram CS, Critchley JA Plasma insulin, growth hormone, cortisol, and central obesity among young Chinese type 2 diabetic patients. *Diabetes Care* 1999; **22**:1450–1457.
40. Reynolds RM, Walker BR, Phillips DIW, Sydall HE, Andrew R, Wood PJ, Whorwood CB Altered control of cortisol secretion in adult men with low birthweight and cardiovascular risk factors. *J Clin Endocrinol Metab* 2001; **86**:245–250.

41. Liu H, Bravata DM, Cabaccan J, Raff H, Ryzen E Elevated late-night salivary cortisol levels in elderly male type 2 diabetic veterans. *Clin Endocrinol (Oxf)* 2005; **63**:642–649.
42. Cameron OG, Thomas B, Tiongco D, Hariharan M, Greden JF Hypercortisolism in diabetes mellitus. *Diabetes Care* 1987; **10**:663.
43. Cameron OG, Kronfol Z, Greden JF, Carroll BJ Hypothalamic-pituitary-adrenocortical activity in patients with diabetes mellitus. *Arch Gen Psych* 1984; **41**:1090–1095.
44. Hudson JI, Hudson MS, Rothschild AJ, Vignati L, Scatzberg AF, Melby JC Abnormal results of dexamethasone suppression tests in nondepressed patients with diabetes mellitus. *Arch Gen Psych* 1984; **41**:1087–1089.
45. Reynolds RM, Sydall HE, Wood PJ, Phillips DIW, Walker BR Elevated plasma cortisol in glucose intolerant men: different responses to glucose and habituation to venepuncture. *J Clin Endocrinol Metab* 2001; **86**:1149–1153.
46. Boyle SH, Surwit RS, Georgiades A, Brummett BH, Helms MJ, Williams RB, Barefoot JC Depressive symptoms, race, and glucose concentrations: the role of cortisol as mediator. *Diabetes Care* 2007; **30**:2484–2488.

Chapter 3
Depression in Older People with Diabetes

Akshya Vasudev and Alan J. Thomas

The Old and Depression

Another chronic illness frequently seen in the older population is depression. The estimates of the prevalence of this condition vary from 1% to 20% [1, 2], rates being much higher for those who are in hospital, those who need home help care and those in long term care. Depression, though, remains poorly diagnosed and subsequently treated and as a result there is a reduced onward referral to specialist services. There may be other reasons for poor rates of uptake of specialist services for treatment and assessment of depression and these might include lack of available specialist services, stigma associated with depression and lack of understanding of the illness. The poor rate of diagnosis and treatment is of concern as depression in older people is associated with a high rate of suicide [3].

Both depression and diabetes are highly prevalent conditions in the aging population. Given this, it is important to determine if these conditions are found together in older people and, if so, what factors might underpin this association. Lastly, it is important to understand the issues that need to be kept in mind when planning treatment and management of both conditions.

A. Vasudev (✉)
Department of Geriatric Psychiatry,
University of Western Ontario and Lawson
Research Institute, London, ON N6A 4G5, Canada

G. Hawthorne (ed.), *Diabetes Care for the Older Patient*,
DOI 10.1007/978-0-85729-461-6_3,
© Springer-Verlag London Limited 2012

Depression and Diabetes in the Older Person

Studies from around the world show that the prevalence of depression and depressive symptoms is much higher in older people with diabetes compared to age matched individuals. Approximately 30% of older people with diabetes have depressive symptoms and 5–10% have major depression [4], compared with rates of 10–15 and 1–3% in the non-diabetic population [5].

The Health, Aging, and Body Composition Study followed up a relatively large cohort of subjects aged 70–79 years in the US (n = 2,552) [6]. There was increased annual incidence of depressed mood in people with diabetes compared to those who did not have diabetes (23.5% vs 19.0%, hazard ratio, 1.31; 95% Confidence Interval (CI), 1.07–1.61). If (type 2) diabetes is well controlled, this increased level of depressive symptoms is not found [7]. A study conducted in a Spanish population who were older than 55 years reported that the prevalence of depression (using a broad criteria for diagnosis) as well as the incidence over 5 years in people with diabetes were 15.4% and 16.5% respectively. Diabetes increased the risk of prevalent (odds ratio [OR] = 1.47; 95% CI: 1.16–1.83) and incident (OR = 1.40; 95% CI: 1.03–1.90) depression. Controlling for potential confounders did not change these findings [8]. Another study in a large rural community of India confirmed that the diagnosis of major depression in the older person was significantly associated with diabetes (OR 2.33; 95% CI 1.15–4.72) after controlling for age, female gender, cognitive impairment and disability status [9]. This was also demonstrated by a study from the middle east that reported that the prevalence of depressive disorder in participants with type 2 diabetes was significantly higher than that of age- and sex-adjusted non diabetic participants (32.1 vs. 16.0%, P < 0.0001) [10].

Recently a study conducted in the UK of patients presenting to primary care found that even though older individuals with diabetes scored high on screening tools for depression including the Patient Health Questionnaire (PHQ), the Beck

Depression Inventory (BDI) and Hospital Anxiety and Depression Scale (HADS), their rate of treatment for depression remained low [11]. This suggests that the older person with diabetes who already has a number of physical and psychosocial changes to grapple with, now is faced with a mental health problem for which he finds it difficult to receive treatment.

Physical Changes Associated with Diabetes

As a person grows old the body undergoes physical decline which manifests as decreases in muscle mass, aerobic capacity, visual and auditory acuity, bone strength and joint flexibility. These changes are more pronounced in the older person who develops diabetes. Furthermore diabetes itself leads to other co-morbidities and complications: these have been covered in other chapters in the book. What is noteworthy is that the more co-morbidities there are, the greater the risk of developing depressive symptoms and major depression. Diabetes itself leads to a number of medical co-morbidities in the elderly that can include falls, urinary incontinence, cognitive impairment, malnutrition as well as depression. Some authors have even gone so far as to consider all these diagnosis as a constellation for a specific geriatric syndrome [12]. In a prospective study of older primary care patients with diabetes who were followed up for five years strong predictors for the development of major depression included having one or more coronary procedures during follow up and the baseline severity of diabetes symptoms [13]. Furthermore, in another study, feeling of 'low well being' increased the risk of development of stroke in the older person with diabetes [14]. In addition abdominal obesity and cardiovascular disease were related to depression in older people with diabetes [15] and women achieving the threshold for major depression as measured by scores on the Centre For Epidemiological Studies Scale for Depression (CES-D) had 24.5% more visceral adipose tissue than those who had lower CES-D scores [16]. A longitudinal cohort study of 4,623 patients with diabetes showed that major depression was associated with increased risk of significant micro and macrovascular complications after adjusting for diabetes severity and self care activity [17].

These studies suggest that there is significant clustering between diabetes, depression and cardiovascular disease in late life. It might be that this association is confounded because of the prevalence of cardiovascular risk factors including obesity and smoking in both the conditions. However, it is also possible that depression and diabetes themselves are 'cardiotoxic' and this explains the strong association. The reader is referred to the literature which has been published in the recent years regarding this relationship which has often been referred to as the vascular depression hypothesis [18–20].

Besides the vascular linkage, attempts have been made to elaborate other neurobiological basis for the association between depression and diabetes. It has been hypothesized that certain neuroendocrine alterations such as the activation of the hypothalamic-pituitary-adrenal (HPA) axis and sympathetic nervous system (SNS) may contribute to both conditions. Additionally, proinflammatory states have been found in both diabetes and depression suggesting another neuruobiological link between these conditions [21]. As of now, these hypotheses have not been adequately tested in a controlled setting..

Functional Disability

Functional impairment manifests frequently in late life because of the physical and psychosocial changes associated with aging. This disability is compounded by the presence of depression and diabetes separately and more so if they are present together. In a large cross sectional sample of adults in the US (n = 30,022), in the National Health Interview Survey respondents were asked about their ability to perform 12 routine tasks without special equipment. These included : ability to walk a quarter of a mile; walk up 10 steps without resting; stand or be on your feet for approximately 2 h; sit for approximately 2 h; stoop, bend or kneel; reach up over your head; use your fingers to grasp or handle small objects; lift or carry a bag full of groceries; push or pull large objects; go out to things like shopping, movies or sporting events; participate in social activities; do things to relax at home or for leisure. The odds of functional disability was 3.00 (95% CI 2.62–3.42) for major depression, 2.42 (2.10–2.79) for diabetes, and 7.15 (4.53–11.28) for diabetes and co-morbid major depression [22]. These odds were found after adjusting for relevant covariates.

Other authors have found that depressive symptoms in the older person with diabetes predisposes them to being almost twice as likely to be physically inactive compared to those who do not have depressive symptoms [23]. Depression in diabetes leads to poor adherence to anti-diabetic medications [24] and people's ability to look after themselves in terms of self care behavior and perceived quality of care is also poorer. They are less likely to engage in leisure time physical activity, smoke more, are less likely to receive opthalmological examination and their flu vaccination [22].

Health Care Costs and Quality of Life

As both depression and diabetes have high individual socio-economic burden costs, it would be expected that in those who have both these illnesses there would be a potentiation of their effects. Indeed in a large meta-analysis hospitalisation rates and hospitalisation costs, frequency and costs of outpatient visits, emergency department visits, medication costs and total healthcare costs were all increased with small to moderate effect sizes in people with diabetes who had co-morbid mental disorders like depression compared to those with diabetes without these problems [25]. Similarly, studies consistently report that quality of life also deteriorates in patients with co-morbid diabetes and depression [26].

The effect of depression on mortality has been investigated in patients with diabetes of old age. Katon et al. [27] found in a longitudinal cohort analysis that minor depressive symptoms were associated with a 1.7 fold increase in mortality and those with major depression had a 2.3 fold increase in risk of mortality over 3 years compared to those who did not have any depressive symptoms. This suggests that depression in the older people with diabetes increases mortality. Perhaps better control of depression and/or diabetes might be expected to lead to a reduction in symptoms and complications emanating from both these serious conditions.

Glycemic Control in Older Patients with Depression and Diabetes

Patients who have both diabetes and depression have been shown to have poorer blood glucose control. This might be related to the patients' own point of view as depressive symptoms might make him less motivated and able to follow dietary advice and poor dietary adherence may result in poor blood glucose levels. This hypothesis has been confirmed in a meta-analysis looking at results from 24 studies conducted in people with Type 1 and Type 2 diabetes [28]. However, data from the older population has not been as consistent [29].

On the other hand, it might be that when people with diabetes and depression interact with health care providers, the providers may set less strict criteria for glycemic control. The providers may perceive that the patient is incapable of achieving appropriate targets for glucose control. Also the diabetes specialist may not feel able to manage the patient's depressive symptoms and this may be compounded by a lack of access to an old age psychiatry specialist. However, currently there is no research evidence to support this suggestion. Whatever the reason, it is known that poor glycemic control predicts a poorer course for depression [30].

Management of Depression in Diabetes in the Older Person

The basic principles of management of depression in the elderly are applicable to the treatment of depressed older people with diabetes. Undeniably, the primary care physician has a key role in diagnosing and treating both these serious conditions. It is also well recognized that the diagnosis of depression in older people remains difficult. Patients frequently deny their depression, often neglecting to recognize their own somatic and cognitive/behavioral depressive symptoms. They underestimate symptom severity and are reluctant to validate the symptoms because of social stigma associated with depression. Also in primary care depressed patients may present with somatic symptoms, which include gastrointestinal, skeletal muscle, and cardiovascular complaints, as opposed to presenting with non-somatic symptoms of depression. Antidepressant pharmacotherapy remains the mainstay of biological treatment of depression. It appears to offer the most benefit to the patient when combined with psychological approaches particularly cognitive and behavioral therapy. When prescribing for older people there should be some consideration of the pharmacokinetic changes related to aging. These might impact on the absorption, distribution, metabolism, and elimination of most of the antidepressants. Polypharmacy because of multiple medical co-morbidities is particularly problematic and amplifies the risk of drug-drug interactions. Nevertheless, antidepressant medications remain as effective in the management of the older depressed person compared to a younger one.

There is a wide array of antidepressant medications available from different classes of antidepressants. The side effect profile of these medications in the older depressed person with diabetes is relatively unknown. The Sequenced Treatment Alternatives to Relieve Depression (STAR*D) study was a large study which enrolled 2,876 outpatients with DSM-IV major depressive disorder from primary and psychiatric care. In this study citalopram was used for a relatively long period of time at usual therapeutic doses (12–14 weeks, 20–60 mg/day). There was no difference in the side effects of citalopram in patients with diabetes compared to non diabetic patients [31].

There is concern that some of the antidepressants themselves are diabetogenic and might impair glycemic control. The evidence base is currently equivocal and the jury is out regarding whether this association is true or not. One publication from Finland included results from a series of nested studies within a large prospective cohort of working-aged men and women including participants with continuing antidepressant medication, severe depression, and those with incident type 2 diabetes mellitus for a mean follow-up of 4.8 years. The 5 year absolute risk of diabetes was 1.1% for non-users of antidepressant medication, 1.7% for individuals treated with 200–399 defined daily doses of antidepressants a year, and 2.3% for those with ≥400 defined daily doses. Antidepressants were associated with weight gain (self reported). Non-users gained 1.4 kg (2.5%) and users of ≥200 defined daily doses gained 2.5 kg (4.3%) (p(trend) < 0.0001) [32]. Mirtazapine, a noradrenergic serotonergic selective uptake inhibitor, has an appetite promoting and sedative effect as part of its profile and this is usually attributed to its histaminergic effects. It is often used in the older depressed population for patients who have significant anorexia and insomnia as part of the depressive syndrome. There are studies to suggest that mirtazapine does cause weight gain because of its ability to increase the appetite. However there are currently no studies reporting its effects on glucose control in the older people with diabetes. In fact, there are no good quality trials to test if antidepressants cause an increase in hyperglycemia in older people with diabetes.

Some studies have been conducted to determine if there are differences in treatment response as well as predictors of response in the depressed diabetic population. One study combined the results of two previously published studies of open label usage of bupropion (n = 93) and sertraline (n = 294). The usage of sertraline predicted poorer treatment response. Other predictors of poor response included the extent of diabetes complication and younger age [33].

Treatment of Depression in Diabetes

Well conducted randomised controlled trials (RCTs) currently offer the best way of assessing the true efficacy and safety of one therapeutic agent compared to another. In a recent review, all published RCTs of treatment of depression in patients suffering from diabetes were compared [34]. The outcome measures included control of depressive symptoms as well as glycemic control. Only four RCTs for depression in diabetes have been published and three of these were conducted in the younger adult population. The results from these trials are reviewed below.

One trial compared the effect of nortriptyline versus placebo in patients with depression and poorly controlled diabetes. Nortriptyline improved depressive symptoms significantly [35] but it also worsened glycemic control. Another trial compared fluoxetine to placebo [36]. Reduction in depression symptoms was significantly greater in patients treated with fluoxetine compared with those receiving placebo and patients on fluoxetine had a better chance of achieving 50% reduction in depression severity, although patients achieving full remission were not significantly different in between the groups. There was a trend for better glycemic control in the fluoxetine group. However, the trial was for a relatively short period of time (8 weeks).

The third RCT compared the continuation of sertraline maintenance treatment over 12 months with placebo [37]. The sertraline group showed a longer depression free interval following recovery from major depression (226 days for subsequent depressive episode in the sertraline group versus 57 days in the placebo group). The beneficial effect of sertraline though was not translated to better glycemic control.

In the only study conducted in the older diabetic population, paroxetine was compared to placebo [38]. The study randomised 49 mildly depressed patients with non-optimally controlled diabetes to a 6 months double-blind treatment with either paroxetine 20 mg/day or placebo. After 3 months of treatment the authors found a statistically significant difference between the two treatment groups in glycosylated haemoglobin (GHbA1c) (mean difference = 0.59%-units [4.1 mmol/mol], p = 0.018) as well as on the SF-36 quality of life score (mean difference = 11.0 points, p = 0.039) favouring paroxetine. When the assessments were repeated at the endpoint of 6 months, these beneficial effects were lost.

Integration Treatment Approaches

Another approach to the management of depressive symptoms in the elderly diabetic patient is to use a combination of eclectic psychotherapy and pharmacological management. In the IMPACT (Improving Mood Promoting Access to Collaborative Treatment) study, elderly patients diagnosed with depression were actively treated by a depression care manager. A subgroup analysis of this trial included diabetic patients (n = 417). A depression care manager, supervised by a psychiatrist and primary care provider, provided support, education, assistance in maintaining the use of antidepressants and problem solving psychotherapy tailored individually to each patient versus usual care. The results from this trial showed improvement in depressive symptoms, overall functioning as well as adherence to recommended exercise in the intervention group [39]. Though there was no suggestion of improvement in glycemic control in the intervention group, as measured by HbA1c levels, the authors accepted the limitation that patients had good glycemic control at baseline, hence power to detect improvements in glycemic control was limited.

Interest has also been growing in collaborative care management of depression and diabetes [40, 41]. A recent study in 214 participants with poorly controlled diabetes, coronary heart disease, or both and coexisting depression was conducted in primary care in the US [42]. Patients were randomized to treatment as usual or the intervention group, in which a medically supervised nurse, working with each patient's primary care physician, provided guideline-based, collaborative care management. Besides receiving support for self-care, patients were allowed changes in medication, as per protocol, for all disease modifying agents (anti-depressant, lipid lowering, insulin and antihypertensives). As compared with controls, patients in the intervention group had statistically significant overall 12 month improvement across glycated hemoglobin levels, LDL cholesterol levels, systolic blood pressure, and depression scores. Patients in the intervention group also were more likely to have one or more adjustments of insulin (P = 0.006), antihypertensive medications (P < 0.001), and antidepressant medications (P < 0.001), and they had better quality of life (P < 0.001) and greater satisfaction with care for diabetes, coronary heart disease, or both (P < 0.001) and with care for depression (P < 0.001). The findings from these two studies suggest that integrative care management might offer additional benefit compared to 'treatment as usual'.

Psychological Treatment Trials

As of yet there has been only one published trial of cognitive behavior therapy (CBT) in depression of late life diabetes [43]. In this study 52 patients were randomized to 10 weeks of diabetes education and CBT for depression or to diabetes education only. At the end point of 6 months, 70% of the patients in the CBT group achieved remission compared with 33% in the education only group. Medical outcomes were also tested. HbA1c deteriorated in the control group (+0.9% [7.5 mmol/mol]) whereas it improved in the CBT group (−0.7% [−5.3 mmol/mol]). Another trial is currently underway in Germany to test efficacy of CBT [44].

Summary

Depression is frequently observed in the older person with diabetes. There are a number of biological and psychosocial factors that underpin this co-morbidity, all of which need to be kept in mind when managing the patient. Vascular risk factors are particularly common in these two conditions; intervention trials addressing these risk factors are sorely needed. Pharmacotherapy with antidepressant medication seems to have the strongest evidence so far in controlling depressive symptoms; however evidence for an improvement in glycemic control is equivocal. Combination of psychological therapy and antidepressants are well accepted and proven treatments of the older depressed population, however there are currently no trials to check the efficacy of this combination in the diabetic older person. Integration treatment approaches are the most intuitive for helping the older depressed person with diabetes achieve better control of both the depressive and diabetic symptoms and this approach fits well with the multi-disciplinary approach for diabetes management.

Practical Points

- The prevalence and incidence of depression is high in older people with diabetes
- There is clustering between depression, diabetes and cardiovascular disease: there might be multidirectional relationship between these disorders
- Depression in late life diabetes is frequently under diagnosed in primary care
- The principles of treating depression are the same for older people with diabetes as for other groups of depressed patients.
- Only one RCT of pharmacologiocal treatment for depression in older people using paroxetine has been published, all other trials are in younger populations
- Integration treatment approaches of managing co-morbid diabetes are intuitive and trials have shown favourable results

References

1. Gurland B, Toner J. Differentiating dementia from nondementing conditions. Adv Neurol. 1983;38:1–17.
2. Masand PS. Depression in long-term care facilities. Geriatrics. 1995 Oct;50 Suppl 1:S16-24.
3. Fiske A, Wetherell JL, Gatz M. Depression in older adults. Annu Rev Clin Psychol. 2009;5:363–89.
4. Black SA. Increased health burden associated with comorbid depression in older diabetic Mexican Americans. Results from the Hispanic Established Population for the Epidemiologic Study of the Elderly survey. Diabetes Care. 1999 Jan;22(1):56–64.

5. Beekman AT, Copeland JR, Prince MJ. Review of community prevalence of depression in later life. Br J Psychiatry. 1999 Apr;174:307–11.

6. Maraldi C, Volpato S, Penninx BW, Yaffe K, Simonsick EM, Strotmeyer ES, et al. Diabetes mellitus, glycemic control, and incident depressive symptoms among 70- to 79-year-old persons: the health, aging, and body composition study. Arch Intern Med. 2007 Jun 11;167(11):1137–44.

7. Golden SH, Lazo M, Carnethon M, Bertoni AG, Schreiner PJ, Diez Roux AV, et al. Examining a bidirectional association between depressive symptoms and diabetes. JAMA. 2008 Jun 18;299(23):2751–9.

8. de Jonge P, Roy JF, Saz P, Marcos G, Lobo A. Prevalent and incident depression in community-dwelling elderly persons with diabetes mellitus: results from the ZARADEMP project. Diabetologia. 2006 Nov;49(11):2627–33.

9. Rajkumar AP, Thangadurai P, Senthilkumar P, Gayathri K, Prince M, Jacob KS. Nature, prevalence and factors associated with depression among the elderly in a rural south Indian community. Int Psychogeriatr. 2009 Apr;21(2):372–8.

10. Shehatah A, Rabie MA, Al-Shahry A. Prevalence and correlates of depressive disorders in elderly with type 2 diabetes in primary health care settings. J Affect Disord. Jun;123(1–3):197–201.

11. Kendrick T, Dowrick C, McBride A, Howe A, Clarke P, Maisey S, et al. Management of depression in UK general practice in relation to scores on depression severity questionnaires: analysis of medical record data. BMJ. 2009;338:b750.

12. Araki A, Ito H. Diabetes mellitus and geriatric syndromes. Geriatr Gerontol Int. 2009 Jun;9(2):105–14.

13. Katon W, Russo J, Lin EH, Heckbert SR, Ciechanowski P, Ludman EJ, et al. Depression and diabetes: factors associated with major depression at five-year follow-up. Psychosomatics. 2009 Nov-Dec;50(6):570–9.

14. Araki A, Murotani Y, Kamimiya F, Ito H. Low well-being is an independent predictor for stroke in elderly patients with diabetes mellitus. J Am Geriatr Soc. 2004 Feb;52(2):205–10.

15. Labad J, Price JF, Strachan MW, Fowkes FG, Ding J, Deary IJ, et al. Symptoms of depression but not anxiety are associated with central obesity and cardiovascular disease in people with type 2 diabetes: the Edinburgh Type 2 Diabetes Study. Diabetologia. Mar;53(3):467–71.

16. Everson-Rose SA, Lewis TT, Karavolos K, Dugan SA, Wesley D, Powell LH. Depressive symptoms and increased visceral fat in middle-aged women. Psychosom Med. 2009 May;71(4):410–6.

17. Lin EH, Rutter CM, Katon W, Heckbert SR, Ciechanowski P, Oliver MM, et al. Depression and advanced complications of diabetes: a prospective cohort study. Diabetes Care. Feb;33(2):264–9.

18. Luijendijk HJ, Stricker BH, Hofman A, Witteman JC, Tiemeier H. Cerebrovascular risk factors and incident depression in community-dwelling elderly. Acta Psychiatr Scand. 2008 Aug;118(2):139–48.

19. Koopmans B, Pouwer F, de Bie RA, Leusink GL, Denollet JK, Pop VJ. Associations between vascular co-morbidities and depression in insulin-naive diabetes patients: the DIAZOB Primary Care Diabetes study. Diabetologia. 2009 Oct;52(10):2056–63.
20. Barnes DE, Alexopoulos GS, Lopez OL, Williamson JD, Yaffe K. Depressive symptoms, vascular disease, and mild cognitive impairment: findings from the Cardiovascular Health Study. Arch Gen Psychiatry. 2006 Mar;63(3):273–9.
21. Champaneri S, Wand GS, Malhotra SS, Casagrande SS, Golden SH. Biological basis of depression in adults with diabetes. Curr Diab Rep. Dec;10(6):396–405.
22. Egede LE, Ellis C, Grubaugh AL. The effect of depression on self-care behaviors and quality of care in a national sample of adults with diabetes. Gen Hosp Psychiatry. 2009 Sep-Oct;31(5):422–7.
23. Koopmans B, Pouwer F, de Bie RA, van Rooij ES, Leusink GL, Pop VJ. Depressive symptoms are associated with physical inactivity in patients with type 2 diabetes. The DIAZOB Primary Care Diabetes study. Fam Pract. 2009 Jun;26(3):171–3.
24. Katon W, Russo J, Lin EH, Heckbert SR, Karter AJ, Williams LH, et al. Diabetes and poor disease control: is comorbid depression associated with poor medication adherence or lack of treatment intensification? Psychosom Med. 2009 Nov;71(9):965–72.
25. Hutter N, Schnurr A, Baumeister H. Healthcare costs in patients with diabetes mellitus and comorbid mental disorders-a systematic review. Diabetologia 2010; 53: 2470–2479 .
26. Goldney RD, Phillips PJ, Fisher LJ, Wilson DH. Diabetes, depression, and quality of life: a population study. Diabetes Care. 2004;27:1066–70.
27. Katon WJ, Rutter C, Simon G, Lin EH, Ludman E, Ciechanowski P, et al. The association of comorbid depression with mortality in patients with type 2 diabetes. Diabetes Care. 2005 Nov;28(11):2668–72.
28. Lustman PJ, Anderson RJ, Freedland KE, de Groot M, Carney RM, Clouse RE. Depression and poor glycemic control: a meta-analytic review of the literature. Diabetes Care. 2000 Jul;23(7):934–42.
29. Trief PM, Morin PC, Izquierdo R, Teresi J, Eimicke JP, Goland R, et al. Depression and glycemic control in elderly ethnically diverse patients with diabetes: the IDEATel project. Diabetes Care. 2006 Apr;29(4):830–5.
30. Lustman PJ, Clouse RE. Treatment of depression in diabetes: impact on mood and medical outcome. J Psychosom Res. 2002 Oct;53(4):917–24.
31. Bryan C, Songer T, Brooks MM, Thase ME, Gaynes B, Klinkman M, et al. Do Depressed Patients With Diabetes Experience More Side Effects When Treated With Citalopram Than Their Counterparts Without Diabetes? A STAR*D Study. Prim Care Companion J Clin Psychiatry. 2009;11(5):186–96.
32. Kivimaki M, Hamer M, Batty GD, Geddes JR, Tabak AG, Pentti J, et al. Antidepressant Medication Use, Weight Gain and Risk of

Type 2 Diabetes Mellitus: A Population-based Study. Diabetes Care 2010; 33:2611–2616

33. Anderson RJ, Gott BM, Sayuk GS, Freedland KE, Lustman PJ. Antidepressant pharmacotherapy in adults with type 2 diabetes: rates and predictors of initial response. Diabetes Care. Mar;33(3):485–9.

34. Petrak F, Herpertz S. Treatment of depression in diabetes: an update. Curr Opin Psychiatry. 2009 Mar;22(2):211–7.

35. Lustman PJ, Griffith LS, Clouse RE, Freedland KE, Eisen SA, Rubin EH, et al. Effects of nortriptyline on depression and glycemic control in diabetes: results of a double-blind, placebo-controlled trial. Psychosom Med. 1997 May-Jun;59(3):241–50.

36. Lustman PJ, Freedland KE, Griffith LS, Clouse RE. Fluoxetine for depression in diabetes: a randomized double-blind placebo-controlled trial. Diabetes Care. 2000 May;23(5):618–23.

37. Lustman PJ, Clouse RE, Nix BD, Freedland KE, Rubin EH, McGill JB, et al. Sertraline for prevention of depression recurrence in diabetes mellitus: a randomized, double-blind, placebo-controlled trial. Arch Gen Psychiatry. 2006 May;63(5):521–9.

38. Paile-Hyvarinen M, Wahlbeck K, Eriksson JG. Quality of life and metabolic status in mildly depressed patients with type 2 diabetes treated with paroxetine: a double-blind randomised placebo controlled 6-month trial. BMC Fam Pract. 2007;8:34.

39. Williams JW, Jr., Katon W, Lin EH, Noel PH, Worchel J, Cornell J, et al. The effectiveness of depression care management on diabetes-related outcomes in older patients. Ann Intern Med. 2004 Jun 15;140(12):1015–24.

40. Ell K, Aranda MP, Xie B, Lee PJ, Chou CP. Collaborative depression treatment in older and younger adults with physical illness: pooled comparative analysis of three randomized clinical trials. Am J Geriatr Psychiatry. 2010 Jun;18(6):520–30.

41. Ell K, Katon W, Xie B, Lee PJ, Kapetanovic S, Guterman J, et al. Collaborative care management of major depression among low-income, predominantly Hispanic subjects with diabetes: a randomized controlled trial. Diabetes Care. 2010 Apr;33(4):706–13.

42. Katon WJ, Lin EH, Von Korff M, Ciechanowski P, Ludman EJ, Young B, et al. Collaborative care for patients with depression and chronic illnesses. N Engl J Med. 2010 Dec 30;363(27):2611–20.

43. Lustman PJ, Griffith LS, Freedland KE, Kissel SS, Clouse RE. Cognitive behavior therapy for depression in type 2 diabetes mellitus. A randomized, controlled trial. Ann Intern Med. 1998 Oct 15;129(8):613–21.

44. Petrak F, Hautzinger M, Plack K, Kronfeld K, Ruckes C, Herpertz S, et al. Cognitive behavioural therapy in elderly type 2 diabetes patients with minor depression or mild major depression: study protocol of a randomized controlled trial (MIND-DIA). BMC Geriatr.10:21.

Chapter 4
Hypoglycaemia and the Older Person

Simon C.M. Croxson

Hypos

Hypoglycaemia is classically defined by Whipple's Triad; it looks like a hypo, plasma glucose level is low, and the patient gets better with treatment [1]. In clinical diabetes, 4.0 mmol/L is taken as the threshold for hypoglycaemia which is often classified as mild if the patient can treat and correct it themselves, or severe if external assistance is required; hypos may however be classified as needing no treatment, treated by patient, treated by external assistance orally, or treated by external assistance parenterally. The glucose level used to define hypoglycaemia is lower for other purposes such as endocrine testing.

Symptoms of Hypoglycaemia in Elderly

As in many illnesses, symptoms of hypoglycaemia may differ between young and old. Jaap et al. [2] demonstrated a wide constellation of symptoms; in 312 diabetic subjects aged 70 years or more on insulin, 102 had had symptomatic

S.C.M. Croxson
Department of Medicine for the Elderly, Ward 17,
University Hospitals Bristol NHS Foundation Trust,
Bristol Royal Infirmary, Marlborough Street,
Bristol, BS2 8HW, UK

G. Hawthorne (ed.), *Diabetes Care for the Older Patient*,
DOI 10.1007/978-0-85729-461-6_4,
© Springer-Verlag London Limited 2012

hypoglycaemia in the prior 2 months with a median of 6 hypos in prior 12 months. They noted that symptoms were less intense in the elderly, and had less autonomic features compared to the young.

Three separate groups of symptoms were noted:

1. Impairment of co-ordination & articulation;
2. More general neuroglycopenic symptoms, such as light-headedness and unsteadiness
3. Autonomic symptoms.

Symptoms included poor concentration, confusion, sweating, trembling, weakness, incoordination, unsteadiness, light headedness, i.e., there was great scope for the symptoms to be attributed to something other than hypoglycaemia such as light headedness being attributed to hypotension.

Matyka et al. [3] studied a group of elderly and young non-diabetic men as their plasma glucose was reduced by an insulin infusion; in the young men, autonomic symptoms occurred at a glucose level of 3.6 mmol/L, and neuroglycopaenic symptoms occurred at 2.8–3.0 mmol/L; in elderly men, sympathetic symptoms occurred at a glucose level of 3.0 mmol/L and neuroglycopaenic symptoms occurred at 2.8–3.0 mmol/L. This suggests that the older person has less time between the development of sympathetic symptoms and neuroglycopaenia than younger subjects. Symptoms were less pronounced in the elderly. On talking to the author, she noted that the older men did not feel quite right, but they could not put their finger on what was wrong. This poorer awareness of hypoglycaemia in elderly had been previously demonstrated in 1995 [4] and a similar study in middle aged and elderly subjects [5] who had diabetes confirmed that hypoglycaemic symptoms were less marked in the older person, and that the older person was much less likely to recognise that they were hypoglycaemic.

A recent study puts hypoglycaemia unawareness in perspective; Munshi et al. [6] used Continuous Glucose Monitoring (mean duration 88 h) on 33 people with diabetes (mean age 75 ± 4.6 years; mean HbA1c $9.4 \pm 1.3\%$ [79 ± 8 mmol/mol]).

77% had type 2 diabetes (T2DM) and 91% were insulin treated. 20 patients had hypos of whom 16 had nocturnal hypos, and 10 had an HbA1c >9% [75 mmol/mol]. In the whole group, the average number of hypoglycaemic episodes was 3.85 per patient. Of the 77 hypoglycaemic episodes, 73 were unrecognized (by either finger-stick monitoring or by symptoms). All patients with hypoglycaemia had at least one unrecognized hypoglycaemic episode, and only 1 of the 32 nocturnal hypos was recognized by patients. So hypoglycaemia in this predominantly insulin treated group was very common, and frequently unrecognised despite high HbA1c levels.

Knowledge of Hypoglycaemia

It has been shown that older folk have extremely poor knowledge about hypoglycaemia [7], and remember events poorly, although family members may recall hypoglycaemic episodes [8]. Hence it is vitally important to see older folk with family members. The prevalence of hypoglycaemia in older people may be grossly underestimated and underappreciated.

Having discussed patient hypoglycaemia unawareness, it is only balanced to consider medical hypoglycaemia unawareness. Hypoglycaemia can present as a fit, transient ischaemic attack, cardiovascular accident, collapse ? cause, "gone off legs", and acute confusion [9], and so hypoglycaemia needs to be considered in the differential diagnosis and recognised by medical staff. Figure 4.1 shows the management of one such patient who had recently commenced 80 mg gliclazide.

As well as medical hypoglycaemia unawareness which has been noted [10], there is medical glycaemia unawareness; in an audit performed by Anna Mason, one of our students, 5 of 45 subjects passed though our department with no estimation of capillary or venous glucose levels; although this is a small sample, the message was clear and a larger sample was not required.

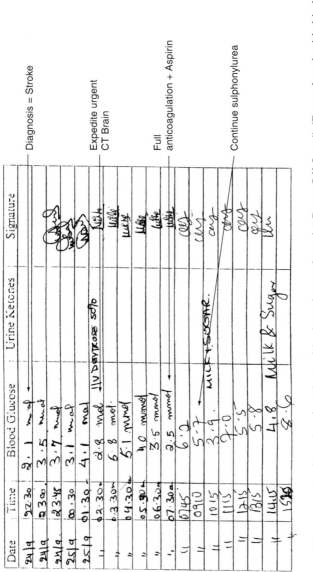

Date	Time	Blood Glucose	Urine Ketones	Signature	
24/9	22.30	2.1 mol			Diagnosis = Stroke
24/9	23.00	3.5 mmol			
24/9	23.45	3.7 mol			
25/9	00.30	3.1 mol			
25/9	01.30	4.1 mol	IV DEXTROSE 50%		Expedite urgent CT Brain
"	02.30~	2.8 mol			
"	03.30~	6.8 mol			
"	04.30~	5.1 mmol			Full anticoagulation + Aspirin
"	05.30~	4.0 mmol			
"	06.30~	3.5 mmol			
"	07.30a	2.5 mmol			
"	0745	6.2			
"	0910	5.7			
"	1015	3.9	MILK + SUGAR.		
"	1115	3.0			Continue sulphonylurea
"	1215	5.5			
"	1315	5.8			
"	1445	4.8	Milk & Sugar		
"	1520	2.6			

FIGURE 4.1 Management of confused patient with slurred speech and "Gone Off Legs" (Reproduced with kind permission of John Wiley and Sons [10])

Epidemiology of Hypoglycaemia

Given that hypoglycaemia is asymptomatic in older folk, the exact incidence and prevalence are not known. Jaap's and Munshi's work showed a median of 6 hypos in 6 months in elderly insulin treated subjects [2], and 66% of older diabetic folk had at least one hypo during 88 h of continuous glucose recording [6] respectively.

Useful figures were given by Shorr et al. [11] in Tennessee Medicaid Enrolees; severe hypoglycaemia (leading to Emergency Dept attendance or hospital admission or death) rates were 1.23/100 patient years on sulfonylurea, 2.76/100 patient years on insulin, and 3.38/100 patient years on insulin plus sulfonylurea. Mean age was 76 years, and although not significant, 25% came from residential care. Two of the 981 hypos proved fatal, and 10 resulted in injury.

Causes and Risk Factors

The commonest cause of hypoglycaemia is diabetes treatment particularly with insulin and sulphonylureas and to a much lesser extent with the prandial glucose regulators (repaglinide and nateglinide). It is disconcerting that one still meets medical practitioners who believe that sulphonylureas do not cause hypoglycaemia.

The traditional quick acting insulins are more likely to produce hypos than the modern rapid acting insulin analogues, and the traditional long acting insulins are more likely to produce hypos than the modern long acting insulin analogues [12].

Among the sulphonylureas, glibenclamide is particularly dangerous with just 2.5 mg reported as killing older folk [13] and chlorpropamide should also be avoided [14,15]. Gliclazide and tolbutamide carry the least risk of hypo with glycaemic control as good as other agents [16]; however, all sulphonylureas can cause significant hypoglycaemia, and my personal

TABLE 4.1 Risk factors for hypoglycaemia – no particular order

Low HbA1c
Recent change hypoglycaemic agent, and type of agent,
Hospitalisation
Co-morbidities; any failure e.g., renal, hepatic, cardiac
Elderly single male
Alcohol
Cognitive impairment
Increasing age

experience is that their duration of effect in the elderly is longer than anticipated. Folk die hypoglycaemic 5 days after their last dose of sulphonylurea [17].

The prandial glucose regulators are safer; repaglinide given at the start of each meal is safer than glibenclamide, but significant hypoglycaemia can still occur, although rare [18]. Nateglinide theoretically should not cause hypoglycaemia and hypos were not seen in the original publications; more recent publications [18] and my clinical experience is that some patients do get mild hypoglycaemic symptoms and plasma glucose levels, which they either safely ignore or easily correct.

Co-prescription of other drugs may alter glycaemic control. There is evidence that ACE inhibitors slightly increase the risk of hypoglycaemia [19, 20]. The evidence is that β blockers do not increase the risk of hypoglycaemia [21], but in practice some patients do state that the β blocker does decrease hypoglycaemia warning and it is very much a case of taking care. Of course, if one stops agents which increase glucose levels e.g., oral glucocorticosteroids or oral β agonists, then hypoglycaemia may ensue and again keeping careful records of previous diabetic control and treatment and adjusting treatment pro-actively is vital.

There are many risk factors for hypoglycaemia [11, 13–15, 17], which are summarised in Table 4.1.

Two interesting points; the risk factors have been known for some time, but are only now appreciated; if one is avoiding metformin because of co-morbidities, the co-morbidities increase the risk of hypoglycaemia.

Moving Targets; a Risk Factor for Hypoglycaemia

Another problem in the elderly is moving targets such as weight change, accommodation change, improvement in glycaemic control. The elderly often lose weight due to co-morbidities or age related loss of appetite which decreases blood glucose and blood pressure i.e., two possible causes of dizzy turns. Thus it is important to proactively spot this, warn patient and carers, and to decrease the hypoglycaemic medication before rather than after hypoglycaemia occurs.

A period of improved glycaemia improves insulin sensitivity and β cell function. This makes the glucose lowering treatment more effective and may lead to hypoglycaemia. Timely review of patients when our treatment has improved glycaemic control is necessary.

It is known that generally, compliance with diet and medication is poor. When people enter residential care, diet is enforced, medication is given but inadequate nutrition and being underweight are common [22]. The subjects also have many risk factors for hypoglycaemia. Thus one would expect significant hypoglycaemia to occur, particularly on first entering residential care. Interestingly, studies show that the elderly resident has fewer hypos and a lower HbA1c than their free range counterpart [23], but one must still be alert to the risk of hypoglycaemia in residents.

Finally, glycaemic targets and priorities change, which can be difficult for our patients to appreciate. Previously patients have generally been striving for tight glycaemic control, and now we are proposing to relax control in light of the possible harmful effects of hypoglycaemia and the patients' age and co-morbidities making tight glycaemic control to avoid of long term complications less relevant.

Driving Down the HbA1c and Measures of Glucose; a Risk Factor for Hypoglycaemia

UKPDS and DCCT [24, 25] both concluded that to improve patient outcomes, one should aim for an HbA1c as low as possible without inducing significant hypoglycaemia, although the hypoglycaemia part often seems to be forgotten. It is clear from DCCT and other studies using insulin or sulphonylurea, that as the HbA1c is driven down, the risk of hypoglycaemia increases.

The HbA1c reflects the average glucose level; in very variable control, a reasonable HbA1c level can disguise significant fluctuations between hypoglycaemia and hyperglycaemia. However, the HbA1c can be altered by factors other than glucose. Variant haemoglobins e.g., persistent HbF [26], have been known for decades to increase the HbA1c, and various abnormal haemoglobins will give spuriously high HbA1c. Age appears to increase the HbA1c by 0.1% [0.86 mmol/mol] per decade [27–29], Afro-Caribbean people seem to have an HbA1c increased by 0.47%–0.65% [3.9–4.8 mmol/mol] [30, 31] and iron deficiency anaemia appears to increase HbA1c by perhaps as much as 4% [32 mmol/mol] [32, 33]. Forthcoming changes to HbA1c results alter the method of reporting, but not the test and these confounding factors will still apply. So the limitations of the HbA1c must be appreciated.

Recent QOF targets released 1st April 2009 set a target of HbA1c under 7.0% [53 mmol/mol]. This may not be appropriate in folk treated with sulphonylurea or insulin given the UK GP database data showing lowest mortality with HbA1c 7.5% [58 mmol/mol] [34].

The frailer older person often has an unremarkable fasting plasma glucose which then rises during the day, this has been documented in the Birmingham Care Home diabetes screening project [35]. Thus if a district nurse is giving a once daily long acting insulin when he/she can, often late morning, the plasma glucose level measured late morning has often risen, but increasing the insulin increases the risk of hypos prebreakfast. Thus home blood glucose monitoring is essential if one wishes to improve glycaemic control safely.

Effects of Hypoglycaemia; Glucose Levels

It is important for patients and carers to know the four things that happen after a hypo, particularly if on insulin:

1. Glucose levels can rise dramatically due to patient's own counter-regulation and their treatment.
2. These high levels generally settle on their own and should not be treated.
3. The person is more likely to go hypo over the next few days.
4. The person is less likely to spot the next hypo.

Thus in patients with extremely variable glucose control, relaxing control, amongst other measures, to avoid hypos is a first step towards optimising insulin treatment.

Effects of Hypoglycaemia; Cognitive Function

In 1994, Gold et al. [36] published a series of five patients with a long history of hypoglycaemia, who developed significant cognitive impairment; the direction of causality was not certain and the authors wondered whether hypoglycaemia could cause permanent cognitive impairment. A further case report [37] carefully assessed a patient with a significant hypoglycaemic episode who was then readmitted with a second severe hypo following which his Abbreviated Mental Test dropped to 5/10 and stayed decreased. The second hypo was due to the patient restarting his sulphonylurea which had been stopped on the first admission. It is important to check for hoarding and to have good communication with GP and family to ensure the offending agent is removed from the home and from the repeat prescription computer system.

A recent study has cast more light on the subject. Whitmer and colleagues examined 16,667 Kaiser Permanente diabetic Californians from 2003 to 2007 [38] who were not known to have dementia or cognitive impairment at the onset of the study (mean age 65 years), and who had been observed for episodes of significant hypoglycaemia from 1980 to 2002. Details of co-morbidities, diabetes and demography were put into a multivariate model. Admission to hospital with one hypo increased risk of future dementia by 1.26 (95% CI 1.1–1.49), and three hypos increased risk by 1.94 (95% CI 1.42–2.64); attending the emergency dept with one hypo increased risk of future dementia by 1.42 and two hypos increased risk by 2.36.

This study has been criticised for under-ascertainment of hypoglycaemia, and a lack of consideration of several other possible confounding factors [39]; the authors accepted that one should be wary of observational data [40], but pointed out that the relationship between hypoglycaemia was strong, graded and did include many confounding variable, so that their study "justifies caution against overtreatment of older patients with diabetes."

Effects of Hypoglycaemia; Cardiac and Mortality

The ACCORD and ADVANCE studies [41, 42] both examined whether improving glycaemic control in T2DM with an intensive 6.5% [48 mmol/mol] HbA1c versus a conventional 7.5% [58 mmol/mol] HbA1c arm would improve outcomes. Both achieved their target HbA1c, although ACCORD did so rapidly. ADVANCE had a non-significant reduction in death and in cardiovascular outcomes, whereas ACCORD had an increase in mortality (HR 1.35; $P=0.04$) and an increase in cardiovascular events (HR 1.22; $P=0.02$).

The cause of the increased mortality in ACCORD has been debated ever since, particularly the role of hypoglycaemia. This has recently been analysed [43] showing that one was less likely to go hypo on conventional target, but that if one did, the mortality rate was higher (see Table 4.2). A significantly lower mortality risk was observed in the intensive arm compared with the standard arm in subjects who experienced at least one hypo needing medical assistance (adjusted HR 0.55, 95% CI 0.31–0.99).

Desouza et al. [44] performed 72 h of continuous glucose monitoring, ECG monitoring and symptom diary in 19 diabetic (T2DM) folk (mean age 58 ± 16 years) with established

TABLE 4.2 Hypoglycaemia and mortality from ACCORD [43]

	Number subjects	Number deaths	Mortality rate (%)
Intensive with hypos	816	53	2.8
Intensive without hypos	4,090	201	1.2
Standard with hypos	256	21	3.7
Standard without hypos	4,832	176	1.0

coronary heart disease on insulin treatment. There were 54 episodes of hypoglycaemia (blood glucose < 3.9 mmol/L) of which 26 were symptomatic, 10 were associated with chest pain, and 6 had electrocardiographic abnormalities. There were 59 episodes of hyperglycaemia (blood glucose > 11.1 mmol/L) with only 1 episode of chest pain and no ECG abnormalities. There were a further 50 episodes when the blood glucose dropped by 5.5 mmol/L over 60 min, and ischaemic symptoms occurred during 9 of these episodes ($P < 0.01$ compared with stable normoglycaemia or hyperglycaemia) and two had electrocardiographic abnormalities. No chest pain or electrocardiographic abnormalities occurred during normal blood glucose. Thus there appears to be an association between episodes of cardiac ischaemia and hypoglycaemia, and it may be that a rapid drop in glucose levels is particularly harmful.

Severe hypoglycaemia in ADVANCE [45] was associated (allowing for multiple confounding factors) with any cause death (HR 2.69, 95% CI 1.97–3.67), cardiovascular death (HR 2.68, 95% CI 1.72–4.19), major macrovascular events (HR 2.88, 95% CI 2.01–4.12), and major microvascular events (HR 1.81, 95% CI 1.19–2.74) (all $P < 0.001$). The conclusion was that the hypoglycaemia was a marker of frailty in ADVANCE and whether frailty or hypoglycaemia was the cause of the adverse events could not be determined. Hypoglycaemia should serve as a warning of future adverse events.

So the coronary events and other adverse outcomes from ACCORD and ADVANCE are probably a mixture of coronary heart disease events precipitated by the hypo, and underlying illness producing hypoglycaemia and adverse outcomes (as previously discussed, any impairment is a risk factor for hypoglycaemia).

UK General Practice observational data [46] shows that compared to metformin and adjusted for confounding variables, sulphonylurea use was associated with greater risk of myocardial infarction and of death. A further UK General Practice observational study showed that in elderly type 2 diabetic subjects taking insulin or sulphonylurea [34], mortality was lowest with an HbA1c of 7.5% [58 mmol/mol]. These studies did not assess hypoglycaemia rate, and are observational making any direction of causality uncertain, but it is plausible that the adverse outcomes relate to hypoglycaemia. The mechanisms whereby hypoglycaemia might cause cardiac events, and myocardial and cerebrovascular ischaemia has recently been expertly reviewed [47].

Effects of Hypoglycaemia; Inpatient Stay

Hypoglycaemia may cause a long stay in hospital in predominantly older people; Johnston et al. collected data on all admissions for hypoglycaemia to Leicester Royal Infirmary for 2 years [48]. The 83 subjects had mean age 76 years (range 51–92 years) and mean duration of hospital stay of 18 days. A study on inpatient hypoglycaemia [49] found that the subjects tended to be elderly (mean age 64 ± 15 years) and that increasing days with hypoglycaemia increased duration inpatient stay, inpatient mortality and 1 year mortality; again the direction of causality is uncertain, but it emphasises the need to watch the older inpatient for hypoglycaemia.

Effects of Hypoglycaemia; Falls and Fractures

It is clear that diabetes is associated with an increased risk of falls and fractures [50] via several possible aetiologies. In Kaiser Permante clients, a lower HbA1c was associated with higher risk of falls [51], but type of medication and presence of hypoglycaemia were not documented. However, a recent study by Schwartz et al. [52] showed that a lower HbA1c on oral agents was not associated with falls, whereas falls were associated with insulin use, which has been seen in other studies [53]. Among Medicaid enrolees, 10 of 981 hypos resulted in injury [11]. Other studies have shown an association between insulin treatment and fractures [54, 55].

So whilst we know that hypoglycaemia causes falls and fractures from our practical experience, and there are associations between low HbA1c and falls and between insulin use and fractures, a clear link between hypoglycaemia and falls or fractures has not been demonstrated in formal studies.

Nocturnal Hypoglycaemia

A comprehensive review by Allen and Frier [56] reported that 50% of severe hypos are nocturnal which may cause low mood or well being next day, cognitive impairment or hypoglycaemia unawareness. So insulin treated diabetic people should test at bedtime, and consider testing at 3:00 a.m. if awake, eat a bedtime snack, and be treated with insulin that has a low risk of overnight hypoglycaemia

Conclusion

Hypoglycaemia in older people is far commoner than generally believed, often unrecognised by patients and healthcare professionals, yet is associated with significant adverse outcomes such as cognitive impairment and death. The direction of causality of this association is still not clear and a formal randomized controlled trial to examine the question would be unethical. Nonetheless, it behoves the healthcare professional to take care (Table 4.3).

TABLE 4.3 Management of hypoglycaemia

Be aware of possibility
If think hypo, test and treat or just treat if cannot test rapidly
Treat with 15 g quick acting CHO e.g., 3 dextrosol tablets, or 100 mL of original Lucozade; carers can smear jam or GlucoGel over gums of unconscious patient
And 15 g long acting CHO e.g., sandwich, biscuits
Patient should be better in 15–20 min; repeat above if necessary
Consider cause of hypo
Ignore high plasma glucose levels after a hypo
Consider glucagon injections for carer administration in type 1 diabetes
Admit patient to hospital if hypo requiring external assistance, particularly if home alone, or on long acting agents

In the older diabetic person, an individualised approach by an experienced knowledgeable clinician is paramount. There are zero randomized controlled trials of glycaemic control in the frail older person; they do not get into the trials.

Practical Points

- Hypoglycaemia in the elderly is more common than appreciated.
- Symptoms of hypoglycaemia in elderly are poorly recognised by patients and healthcare professionals
- If using a sulphonylurea or insulin:
  - Ensure adequate diet; The Nutrition Advisory Group for Elderly People of the British Dietetic Association (www.bda.uk.com) produce excellent diet sheets.
  - Use the agent with lowest hypoglycaemia risk
  - Ensure patient, family and carers are educated about hypoglycaemia

- If avoiding metformin because of contraindications, these contraindications increase risk of hypoglycaemia.
- Anticipate hypoglycaemia in subjects entering residential care, or losing weight.
- Ask both patient, family and carers about "funny turns" and possible hypoglycaemia.
- Good communication between patient, family, carers and healthcare professionals is essential to prevent recurrence of hypoglycaemia.

References

1. American Diabetes Association Workgroup On Hypoglycemia Defining and reporting hypoglycemia in diabetes. Diabetes Care, 2005;28:1245–1249.
2. Jaap AJ, Jones GC, McCrimmon RJ, Deary IJ, Frier BM. Perceived symptoms of hypoglycaemia in elderly Type 2 diabetic patients treated with insulin. Diabet. Med. 1998;15:398–401.
3. Matyka K, Evans M, Lomas J, Cranston I, Macdonald I, Amiel SA. Altered hierarchy of protective responses against severe hypoglycaemia in normal ageing in healthy men. Diabetes Care 1997; 20:135–141.
4. Brierley EJ, Broughton DL, James OF, Alberti KG. Reduced awareness of hypoglycaemia in the elderly despite an intact counter-regulatory response. QJM. 1995;88:439–45.
5. Bremer JP, Jauch-Chara K, Hallschmid M, Schmid S, Schultes B. Hypoglycemia unawareness in older compared with middle-aged patients with Type 2 diabetes. Diabetes Care 2009;32:1513–1517.
6. Munshi MN, Segal AR, Suhl E, Staum E; Desrochers L, Sternthal, Giusti J, McCartney R, Lee Y, Bonsignore P, Weinger K. Frequent Hypoglycemia Among Elderly Patients With Poor Glycemic Control. Arch Intern Med. 2011;171:362–364.
7. Thomson FJ, Masson EA, Leeming JT, Boulton AJ Lack of knowledge of symptoms of hypoglycaemia by elderly diabetic patients. Age Ageing. 1991;20:404–6.
8. Heller S, Chapman J, McCloud J, Ward J. Unreliability of reports of hypoglycaemia by diabetic patients. BMJ. 1995;310:440.
9. McAulay V, Deary IJ, Frier BM. Symptoms of hypoglycaemia in people with diabetes. Diabet Med. 2001;18:690–705.
10. Croxson SCM. Hypoglycaemia, cognition and the older person with diabetes. Pract Diab Int 2010;27:219–220.

11. Shorr RI, Ray WA, Daugherty JR, Griffin MR: Incidence and risk factors for serious hypoglycaemia in older persons using insulin or sulfonylureas. Arch Intern Med 1997;157:1681–1686.

12. Gough SC. A review of human and analogue insulin trials. Diabetes Res Clin Pract. 2007;77:1–15.

13. Aslpund K, Wihilm B-E, Lithner F. Glibenclamide associated hypoglycaemia; a report on 57 cases. Diabetologia 1983;24:412–417.

14. Stahl M, Berger W. Higher incidence of severe hypoglycaemia leading to hospital admission in type 2 diabetic patients treated with long-acting versus short-acting sulphonylureas. Diabet Med 1999;16:586–90.

15. Shorr RI, Ray WA, Daugherty JR, Griffin MR. Individual sulfonylureas and serious hypoglycemia in older people. J Am Geriatr Soc. 1996;44:751–5.

16. Harrower AD, Wong C. Comparison of secondary failure rate between three second generation sulphonylureas. Diabetes Res. 1990;13(1):19–21.

17. Croxson S, Chapter 19: Diabetes mellitus & common endocrine conditions in the elderly. In Crome P, Ford G, (Eds) Drugs & the older population. London: Imperial College Press, 2000, 453–531.

18. Black C, Donnelly P, McIntyre L, Royle PL, Shepherd JP, Thomas S. Meglitinide analogues for type 2 diabetes mellitus. Cochrane Database of Systematic Reviews 2007, Issue 2. Art. No.: CD004654. DOI: 10.1002/14651858.CD004654.pu3.

19. Morris AD, Boyle DI, McMahon AD et al ACE inhibitor use is associated with hospitalization for hypoglycemia in patients with diabetes. Diabetes Care 1997;20:1363–7.

20. Herings RM, de Boer A, Stricker BH, Leufkens HG, Porsius A. Hypoglycaemia associated with use of inhibitors of angiotensin converting enzyme. Lancet. 1995;345:1195–8.

21. A H Barnett, D Leslie, and P J Watkins. Can insulin-treated diabetics be given beta-adrenergic blocking drugs? B M J. 1980;280:976–978.

22. Benbow SJ, Hoyte R, Gill GV. Institutional dietary provision for diabetic patients. QJM. 2001;94:27–30.

23. Mooradian AD, Osterweil D, Petrasek D, Morley JE. Diabetes mellitus in elderly nursing home patients. A survey of clinical characteristics and management. J Am Geriatr Soc. 1988;36:391–6.

24. UK Prospective Diabetes Study (UKPDS) Group. Intensive blood-glucose control with sulphonylureas or insulin compared with conventional treatment and risk of complications in patients with type 2 diabetes (UKPDS 33): Lancet 1998;352:837–853.

25. The Diabetes Control and Complications Trial Research Group: The effect of intensive treatment of diabetes on the development and progression of long-term complications in insulin-dependent diabetes mellitus. N Engl J Med1993;329:977–986.

26. Paisey RB, Read R, Palmer R, and Hartog M. Persistent fetal haemoglobin and falsely high glycosylated haemoglobin levels. BMJ (Clin Res Ed). 1984;289:279–280.

27. Simon D, Senan C, Garnier P, Saint-Paul M, Papoz L. Epidemiological features of glycated haemoglobin A1c-distribution in a healthy population. The Telecom Study. Diabetologia. 1989;32:864–9.

28. Kilpatrick ES, Dominiczak MH, Small M. The effects of ageing on glycation and the interpretation of glycaemic control in Type 2 diabetes. QJM, 1996;89:307–12.

29. Pani LN, Korenda L, Meigs JB, Driver C, Chamany S, Fox CS, Sullivan L, D'Agostino RB, Nathan DM. Effect of aging on A1C levels in individuals without diabetes: evidence from the Framingham Offspring Study and the National Health and Nutrition Examination Survey 2001–2004. Diabetes Care. 2008;31:1991–6.

30. Ziemer DC, Kolm P, Weintraub WS, Vaccarino V, Rhee MK, Twombly JG, Narayan KM, Koch DD, Phillips LS. Glucose-independent, black-white differences in hemoglobin A1c levels: a cross-sectional analysis of 2 studies. Ann Intern Med. 2010;152: 770–7.

31. Kirk JK, D'Agostino RB Jr, Bell RA, Passmore LV, Bonds DE, Karter AJ, Narayan KM. Disparities in HbA1c levels between African-American and non-Hispanic white adults with diabetes: a meta-analysis. Diabetes Care. 2006;29:2130–6.

32. Brooks AP, Metcalfe J, Day JL, Edwards MS. Iron deficiency and glycosylated haemoglobin A. Lancet. 1980;2:141.

33. Davis RE, McCann VJ, Nicol DJ. Influence of iron-deficiency anaemia on the glycosylated haemoglobin level in a patient with diabetes mellitus. Med J Aust. 1983;1:40–1.

34. Currie CJ, Peters JR, Tynan A, Evans M, Heine RJ, Bracco OL, Zagar T, Poole CD. Survival as a function of HbA(1c) in people with type 2 diabetes: a retrospective cohort study. Lancet. 2010;375: 481–9

35. Croxson SCM. Chapter 3; Screening for diabetes. In Sinclair AJ, (Ed). Diabetes in old age (3nd edition). Chichester; John Wiley & Sons; 2009; pp 21–40.

36. Gold AE, Deary IJ, Jones RW, O'Hare JP, Reckless J, Frier BM. Severe deterioration in cognitive function and personality in five patients with longstanding diabetes: a complication of diabetes or a consequence of treatment. Diabet Med 1994;11:499–505.

37. Croxson S, McConvey R, Molodynski L. Severe hypoglycaemia & cognitive impairment. Pract Diab Int 2001;18:315–316.

38. Whitmer RA, Karter AJ, Yaffe K, Quesenberry CP Jr, Selby JV. Hypoglycemic episodes and risk of dementia in older patients with type 2 diabetes mellitus. JAMA. 2009;301:1565–1572.

39. Graveling AJ, Frier BM. Dementia and hypoglycemic episodes in patients with type 2 diabetes mellitus. JAMA. 2009 Aug 26; 302:843.

40. Whitmer RA, Karter AJ, Selby JV. Dementia and hypoglycemic episodes in patients with Type 2 diabetes mellitus—Reply. JAMA. 2009;302:843–844.
41. The Action to Control Cardiovascular Risk in Diabetes Study Group. Effects of intensive glucose-lowering in type 2 diabetes. New Engl J Med 2008;358:2545–59.
42. The ADVANCE Collaborative Group. Intensive blood glucose control and vascular outcomes in patients with type 2 diabetes. N Engl J Med 2008;358:2560–72.
43. Bonds DE, Miller ME, Bergenstal RM, Buse JB, Byington RP, Cutler JA, Dudl RJ, Ismail-Beigi F, Kimel AR, Hoogwerf B, Horowitz KR, Savage PJ, Seaquist ER, Simmons DL, Sivitz WI, Speril-Hillen JM, Sweeney ME. The association between symptomatic, severe hypoglycaemia and mortality in type 2 diabetes: retrospective epidemiological analysis of the ACCORD study. BMJ. 2010;340:b4909. doi: 10.1136/bmj.b4909.
44. Desouza C, Salazar H, Cheong B, Murgo J, Fonseca V. Association of hypoglycemia and cardiac ischemia: a study based on continuous monitoring. Diabetes Care. 2003;26:1485–9.
45. Zoungas S, Patel A, Chalmers J, de Galan BE, Li Q, Billot L, Woodward M, Ninomiya T, Neal B, MacMahon S, Grobbee DE, Kengne AP, Marre M, Heller S, for the ADVANCE Collaborative Group. Severe hypoglycemia and risks of vascular events and death. N Engl J Med 2010;363:1410–1418
46. Tzoulaki I, Molokhia M, Curcin V, Little MP, Millett CJ, Ng A, Hughes RI, Khunti K, Wilkins MR, Majeed A, Elliott P. Risk of cardiovascular disease and all cause mortality among patients with type 2 diabetes prescribed oral antidiabetes drugs: retrospective cohort study using UK general practice research database. BMJ. 2009;339:b4731. doi: 10.1136/bmj.b4731.
47. Wright RJ, Frier BM. Vascular disease and diabetes: is hypoglycaemia an aggravating factor? Diabetes Metab Res Rev. 2008;24:353–63.
48. Johnston V, Howe J, Davies M. Hospital admission secondary to hypoglycaemia in type 2 diabetes. J Diabetes Nursing 2002;6:51–55
49. Turchin A, Matheny ME, Shubina M, Scanlon JV, Greenwood B, Pende. Hypoglycemia and clinical outcomes in patients with diabetes hospitalized in the general ward. Diabetes Care. 2009; 32:1153–7.
50. Mayne D, Stout NR, Aspray TJ. Diabetes, falls and fractures. Age Ageing. 2010;39:522–5.
51. Nelson JM, Dufraux K, Cook PF. The relationship between glycemic control and falls in older adults. J Am Geriatr Soc. 2007; 55:2041–4.
52. Schwartz AV, Vittinghoff E, Sellmeyer DE, Feingold KR, de Rekeneire N, Strotmeyer ES, Shorr RI, Vinik AI, Odden MC, Park SW, Faulkner KA, Harris TB; Health, Aging, and Body Composition Study. Diabetes-related complications, glycemic control, and falls in older adults. Diabetes Care. 2008;31:391–6.

53. Berlie HD, Garwood CL. Diabetes medications related to an increased risk of falls and fall-related morbidity in the elderly. Ann Pharmacother. 2010;44:712–7.
54. Schwartz AV, Sellmeyer DE, Ensrud KE, Cauley JA, Tabor HK, Schreiner PJ, Jamal SA, Black DM, Cummings SR; Study of Osteoporotic Features Research Group. Older women with diabetes have an increased risk of fracture: a prospective study. J Clin Endocrinol Metab. 2001;86:32–38.
55. Monami M, Cresci B, Colombini A, Pala L, Balzi D, Gori F, Chiasserini V, Marchionni N, Rotella CM, Mannucci E. Bone fractures and hypoglycemic treatment in type 2 diabetic patients: a case-control study. Diabetes Care. 2008;31:199–203.
56. Allen KV, Frier BM. Nocturnal hypoglycemia: clinical manifestations and therapeutic strategies toward prevention. Endocr Pract. 2003;9:530–43.

Chapter 5
Cardiovascular Risk, Glucose and Targets for Management of Diabetes in Older People

Gillian Hawthorne and Alison J. Yarnall

Older people make up a large proportion of people with diabetes, and although there is much guidance for the treatment of people with type 2 diabetes, these do not take into account the real situation in the elderly such as co-morbidities and frailty. Indeed, frail elderly are routinely excluded from large clinical trials, where cardiovascular risk, hypertension and risk of death are so much higher. This chapter discusses current trial evidence for cardiovascular risk, glucose and targets for management of diabetes in older people, allowing for the heterogeneous nature of this group and offering some practical guidance for practising clinicians in this difficult area.

Although there are many guidelines for the management of type 2 diabetes [National Institute for Health and Clinical Excellence (NICE), Scottish Intercollegiate Guidelines Network (SIGN), American Diabetes Association (ADA)], most of these guidelines make no concession for the effect of age and frailty. Diabetes is increasing in prevalence in the over 60s and this group are at particular risk of repeated hospital admission [1].

Within the over 60 years group there is heterogeneity and a wide range of varying physiological profiles. The age at which diabetes was diagnosed and its duration impacts

G. Hawthorne (✉)
Newcastle Diabetes Centre, The Newcastle upon tyne Hospitals,
NHS Foundation Trust, Campus for Ageing and Vitality,
NE46BE, Newcastle upon Tyne, UK

G. Hawthorne (ed.), *Diabetes Care for the Older Patient*,
DOI 10.1007/978-0-85729-461-6_5,
© Springer-Verlag London Limited 2012

on ongoing care. While older people tend to have normal hepatic glucose output, ageing is associated with declining pancreatic islet cell function and lower insulin levels. Lean older people secrete markedly less insulin in response to a glucose load [2]. Those who develop type 2 diabetes in old age are more likely to have near normal fasting glucose levels but significant post-prandial hyperglycaemia [3, 4]. Factors such as medications that can induce hyperglycaemia, reduced physical activity and concomitant infections may also predispose this population to higher glucose levels. In non-diabetic subjects, insulin secretion declines at a rate of around 0.7% per year with age; the figure is double in those with impaired glucose tolerance [5]. Lastly, a reduction in intracellular body water, increase in body fat and a reduction in muscle mass as part of normal ageing can mean a progression to insulin resistance [6]. The physiology of diabetes and ageing is important as it affects diagnosis and treatment of the condition in the older person.

Cardiovascular Risk

Coronary heart disease is reported to be declining in the Western world [7], but in people with diabetes there still is a twofold higher mortality from coronary heart disease. Data from Norway shows that mortality from coronary heart disease declined in people with diabetes between two population surveys in 1984–1986 and 1995–1997. In this population study in people with diabetes, the mortality rate fell from 15.20 in the 1980s to 1.71 in the 1990s for those aged 60–69 years. In those aged 70–79, the mortality rate fell from 28.15 to 11.83 over that 10 year period, and for those over 80 from 51.63 to 24.5. This highlights the increased burden of coronary heart disease in older age bands.

Similarly, a US study following the natural history of people with newly diagnosed type 2 diabetes in the over 65 years compared outcomes to those without diabetes [8]. During a 10 year follow up, those with diabetes had an excess of mortality of 9.7% compared with the non diabetic population. Heart failure was diagnosed in 57.6% of those with diabetes compared to 34.1% of controls. At 10 years 91.8% of those with diabetes had an adverse complication compared to 72% in the non diabetic group. Studies have shown that predictors of mortality in older people with diabetes mellitus include albuminuria and a history of congestive heart failure (CHF) [9, 10]. In a comparable analysis, participants in the Cardiovascular Health Study, a prospective, longitudinal observational study of 5,888 adults, who were 65 years or above were followed from 1989 to 2001 [11]. This cohort was limited to people living at home. Older adults with diabetes were at a very high absolute risk of death from cardiovascular causes (4–5% per year). Insulin treated participants had higher total mortality than those treated by oral glucose lowering therapy.

Although control of hyperglycaemia is important for older people with diabetes, a greater reduction in morbidity and mortality might result from control of cardiovascular risk factors than glycaemic control [12]. There is clinical evidence that approximately 8 years must elapse before benefits of glycaemic control are reflected in the reduction of microvascular complications [13, 14] whereas control of cardiovascular risk factors of blood pressure and lipids show benefit within 2 years [15–17].

The lack of significance of diabetes control was illustrated in an observational study of a cohort of intensively managed older people aged over 65 years with type 2 diabetes (mean HbA1c 6.8% [51 mmol/mol]) and blood pressure (BP) 136/74. The participants were followed for 3 years had a mortality rate of 2.9% per year. This was comparable to the age and sex matched general population [18]. The major cause of death was malignancy, followed by stroke then myocardial infarction (MI). This study also noted that systolic BP below 125 mmHg was not a good prognostic sign and that HbA1c in the range 5.56–8.3% [38–67 mmol/mol] did not impact on outcome.

Most older adults with diabetes mellitus have at least one other chronic disease. Diabetes is more likely to be associated with medium term mortality than co-morbidity [19]. Frail older adults with diabetes are more than twice as likely to have a complication of diabetes than those who are not frail, and their median life expectancy is 23 months. This study also found that diabetes was a significant predictor of death, although frailty was the most significant predictor of mortality. A systematic review of randomised controlled trials that study diabetes and co-morbidities in older adults identified a large pool of studies. However, most were small studies focussing on cardiovascular outcomes and few addressed non cardiovascular co-morbidity [20]. The limited life expectancy of frail older people emphasises the importance of recognising frailty and individualising care [19]. Care should therefore be individualised based on frailty, life expectancy, patient and/or carer preference and co morbid conditions.

Glucose Control

While diabetes is recognised as a major risk factor for cardiovascular disease, the optimal target for glucose control as measured by HbA1c is still debated. The landmark study of the UK Prospective Diabetes Study Group (UKPDS) highlighted that an HbA1c of < 7% [53 mmol/mol] compared to 7.9% [63 mmol/mol] resulted in a relative risk reduction of microvascular complications by 25% over a 10 year period, but there was no significant impact on the risk of myocardial infarction (MI) or all-cause mortality [21]. HbA1c treated to 8% [64 mmol/mol] for a further 10 years, however, resulted in a significant relative risk reduction in myocardial infarction and death from any cause [22]. This so called 'legacy' effect has led clinicians to emphasise the importance of tight glucose control in the initial stages of diabetes diagnosis in order to reduce the burden of microvascular complications, MI and death in later years. However, the relevance of this to newly diagnosed elderly frail patients with a life expectancy of less than 10 years is doubtful.

Observational data from the UKPDS show that if glycaemia has a role in macroangiopathy, the maximum benefit from reducing HbA1c by 1% [8.6 mmol/mol] over 10 years is a 14% reduction in myocardial infarction and a 12% reduction in stroke [13]. The benefits achieved from tight glycaemic control require about 8 years to prevent microvascular complications and are associated with an increased risk of hypoglycaemia. Intervention studies with statins and anti-hypertensive drugs have benefits which are double this, and they may be correlated with fewer side effects. A number of trials on glucose control in older patients and macrovascular disease are now explored.

In the ADVANCE trial, over 11,000 participants achieved a HbA1c of 6.5% [48 mmol/mol] in the intensively treated group versus 7.3% in the standard control group over a median of 5 years of follow-up [23]. The mean age at baseline was 66 years, and all had a history of major macrovascular or microvascular disease or at least one other risk factor for vascular disease. The intensively treated group were commenced on a sulphonylurea and their treatment progressively increased with or without the addition of metformin, thiazolidinediones, acarbose or insulin. Although there was a statistically significant difference in nephropathy in the intensively treated participants (4.1% versus 5.2%), there was no reduction in macrovascular events. Those treated intensively were more likely to be hospitalised (44.9% versus 42.8%) and were at risk of severe hypoglycaemia (rate of severe hypoglycaemia 2.7% compared with 1.5%).

Similarly the ACCORD trial failed to show a benefit on major cardiovascular outcomes in those intensively treated with glucose-lowering agents. 10,251 patients with a mean age of 62 years were randomised to receive intensive therapy with a target HbA1c of <6% [42 mmol/mol], or standard therapy (target 7.0–7.9% [53–63 mmol/mol]) [24]. At follow-up, HbA1c was 6.4% [46 mmol/mol] and 7.5% [58 mmol/mol], respectively. Those in the intensively treated arm had significantly higher rates of severe hypoglycaemia (10.5% versus 3.5%), weight gain (mean weight gain 3.5 kg compared with 0.4 kg at 3 years) and fluid retention (70.1% of patients versus 66.8%). Although the rate of non-fatal MI was decreased in those intensively treated, the rate of death from cardiovascular cause was higher, and there was an absolute increase in mortality of 1% in the treatment group. This higher rate of death together with the unacceptably high levels of hypoglycaemia led to the conclusion that tight glycaemic control offers no benefit in terms of macrovascular disease and significantly increases the risk of severe hypoglycaemia.

Comparable results were found in the Veterans Affairs Diabetes Trial (VADT) published following the above named trials [25]. 1,791 largely overweight, male military veterans with a mean age of 60.4 years who were at high risk of cardiovascular disease and with poorly controlled diabetes (mean HbA1c at baseline 9.4% [79 mmol/mol]) were randomised to receive either intensive or standard glucose control. The aim of the intensive-therapy group was an absolute reduction in HbA1c of 1.5% [12.9 mmol/mol]. Primary outcome was time to first major cardiovascular event, and secondary outcomes included microvascular complications. Participants in the intensive-treatment group were started on maximal doses of dual oral therapy, and insulin was added if they failed to reach an HbA1c of less than 6% [42 mmol/mol]. After 6 years of follow-up, blood pressure, lipid levels and smoking use fell in both groups, with an increase in anti-platelet and statin prescribing, which almost certainly accounted for the fewer cardiovascular events than were predicted. Although the goal of intensive-therapy was met, with a median HbA1c of 6.9% [52 mmol/mol] (versus 8.4% [68 mmol/mol] in the standard therapy group), there were no significant differences in the primary or secondary outcomes between the groups. Those treated intensively had a significant increase in episodes of severe hypoglycaemia (P<0.001). Again it was concluded that intensive glucose control does not reduce cardiovascular events, has negligible effects on microvascular outcomes and indeed may cause considerable morbidity in terms of episodes of hypoglycaemia.

From these three recent major trials, we can conclude that intensive glucose control (HbA1c < 7% [53 mmol/mol]) does not reduce cardiovascular risk and is likely to be harmful for our elderly patients with a high risk of hypoglycaemia. Hypoglycaemia is the commonest metabolic complication in the elderly, and causes substantial morbidity and mortality in terms of stroke, cardiac ischaemia and arrhythmias [26]. It also may affect confidence and compliance with medications. Additionally, emerging evidence suggests that hypoglycaemia severe enough to require a hospital admission or attendance to an emergency department is a risk factor for the development of dementia, especially in those with multiple episodes [27]. Despite the evidence above, many of our older patients remain tightly controlled on multiple medications. Although hypoglycaemia may cause significant health issues, hyperglycaemia is also an important source of morbidity, and is a risk factor for the development of sepsis, dehydration and hyperglycaemic hyperosmolar state. This U-shaped association for mortality at both low and high mean HbA1c was demonstrated in a recent trial published in The Lancet [28]. Two cohorts of people with type 2 diabetes who were 50 years and older were followed for a mean of 4.5 years and 4.4 years. Mean age overall was 63.6. In both cohorts, HbA1c values in the lowest decile (median 6.4% [46 mmol/mol]) were associated with a heightened risk for all cause mortality for all patients. HbA1c in the highest decile (mean HbA1c 10.5% [91 mmol/mol]) was also associated with an increased risk of all cause mortality. HbA1c of approximately 7.5% [58 mmol/mol] was associated with lowest all-cause mortality and lowest progression to large vessel disease. A reduction or increase in HbA1c away from this mean value enhanced the risk of adverse events, and adds weight to the evidence above that intensive glucose control is not safe in older patients, but also that marked hyperglycaemia should be avoided.

What about glycaemic control and other markers of morbidity in the elderly? Previous studies have shown that falls, a common 'Geriatric Giant,' occur in 39% of older diabetic subjects, with further risk factors including female sex, advanced age and poor diabetes control (HbA1c > 7% [53 mmol/mol]) [29]. These falls are probably multifactorial and contributing factors are likely to include orthostatic hypotension secondary to autonomic dysfunction and medications, peripheral neuropathy, gait disorder and reduced vision. Diabetes itself is thought to increase the risk of fracture [30], and the relationship between glucose control and falls has also been studied. Achieving a HbA1c of less than 6.0% [42 mmol/mol] in older diabetic people (mean age 73.6 years) with oral hypoglycaemic agents was not associated with falls but for those people on insulin, a HbA1c less than 6% [42 mmol/mol] was associated with falling (odds ratio (OR) 4.36) compared with a HbA1c of >8% [64 mmol/mol] [31]. Contrary to the study by Tilling et al., poor glycaemic control was not associated with falling, and the study group postulated that hypoglycaemic episodes may have contributed to this excess falls risk in the insulin-treated group.

There is a lack of clinical trial data evaluating the benefits of long term intensive glucose control in older people, especially those with multiple co-morbid conditions. The benefit of tight glycaemic control (HbA1c less than 6.5% [48 mmol/mol] compared with HbA1c less than 7.0% [53 mmol/mol]) was assessed in an observational study of 2,613 patients with type 2 diabetes in Italy. Patients with low to moderate (but not high co-morbidity) with tight glucose control had a lower risk of cardiovascular events over 5 years [32]. Co morbidity was measured using the Total Illness Burden Index, which assessed the co morbid conditions atherosclerotic heart disease, lung disease, congestive heart failure, arthritis, genitourinary disease, vision loss, gastrointestinal conditions, and foot disease. Patients with high co-morbidity were older (64.3 years vs. 61.7), more likely to have never smoked, had higher BMIs, longer duration of diabetes (11.9 vs. 9.7 years) and had higher HbA1c levels (7.4% [57 mmol/mol] vs. 7.2% [55 mmol/mol]). Those patients with high co-morbidity had no association between attaining HbA1c targets of 6.5% [48 mmol/mol] or less and experiencing a cardiovascular event during the 5 year follow up, that is, those frailer patients with multiple co-morbidities with intensive blood glucose control did not have a reduction in cardiovascular events. Co-morbidity is an important consideration when individualising glucose lowering treatment for older people with type 2 diabetes.

A decision analysis using an integration of multiple prediction models from the fields of diabetes and geriatrics was used to estimate the net benefits of treating older people aged 60–80 years with various life expectancies to a target HbA1c of 7% [53 mmol/mol] compared to 7.9% [63 mmol/mol]. [33]. The benefits of tight control amounted to an additional 51–116 additional quality adjusted days, which decreased with increased age and reduced life expectancy. These findings suggested that HbA1c targets should be relaxed for older people with co-morbid illness. In individuals with no co-morbid illness, the expected quality adjusted benefits of intensive glucose control was 106 days, and this decreased to 52 days at 75–79 years. A mortality index was developed which had a total score of 26 and was scored on co-morbid illness and functional impairment, with each co morbidity or functional impairment contributing 1 or 2 points to the index score. As this score increased, life expectancy decreased and quality adjusted benefits fell. For patients aged 60–64 years with a duration of diabetes 10–15 years, the expected benefits decreased from 116 to 8 days if 8 index points were present. Limited life expectancy was shown to be an important determinant of the expected benefit of intensive glucose treatment compared with moderate glucose treatment, even among people with longstanding diabetes. The authors suggest that 5 years of life expectancy is an acceptable threshold for identifying older people who are unlikely to benefit from intensive control as they would gain only 20 quality adjusted days with intensive treatment. For patients aged 60–64 with a combination of four long-standing co-morbid conditions and a life expectancy of less than 5 years: they gained only 8–13 additional quality adjusted days from intensive glucose control.

Diabetes goals and glycaemic targets should therefore be carefully tailored to individual older patients, taking into account co-morbidities, frailty, life expectancy, functional impairment, likely adherence to treatment, falls risk and risk of hypoglycaemia.

Practical Recommendations

Targets for Glycaemic Control

- NICE guidance (which is not age specific) suggests that people with type 2 diabetes treated with diet and up to two oral glucose-lowering therapies at maximum dosage should have a HbA1c less than 6.5% [48 mmol/mol] [34].
- Those on insulin therapy and triple oral medication should aim for HbA1c less than 7.5% [58 mmol/mol].
- The target HbA1c for older people recommended by the American Geriatric Society is 8.0% [64 mmol/mol],but the European Diabetes Working Group for Older People [35] sets this target at 8% [64 mmol/mol] or less for older people with frailty or advanced disease, or <7% [53 mmol/mol] for those with minimal co-morbidities.

Oral Glucose Lowering Treatment

Metformin has the advantage of reducing the risk of myocardial infarction and hypoglycaemia, but in old frail adults it might worsen age related changes in caloric intake. Gastrointestinal side-effects are common and dose-dependent, and may limit its use. In the USA, metformin is contraindicated for those over 80 years, but the European Diabetes Working Party for Older People guidelines for type 2 diabetes [35] state that age per se is not a contraindication to its use. Metformin is contraindicated if eGFR is 30 or less, and in conditions which may predispose to lactic acidosis such as sepsis, acute dehydration, hepatic dysfunction and in acute coronary events. Consequently, many older adults may have contra-indications or intolerances that preclude the use of metformin.

Sulphonylureas such as gliclazide are indicated in older people as first line if body mass index (BMI) is between 22 and 25 kg/m^2. Older people are more likely to develop hypoglycaemia on sulphonylureas, and the European Diabetes Working Party guidelines for type 2 diabetes do not recommend glibenclamide for those aged over 70 due to the unacceptably high risk of hypoglycaemia. The weight gain associated with sulphonylurea treatment may be advantageous in some elderly frail patients. The risk of hypoglycaemia may be less with meglitinides such as repaglinide [36], which like sulphonylureas work as insulin secretagogues. Their rapid onset of action and shorter half lives mean that they are a practical choice for the frailer elderly with erratic eating habits.

There has been much controversy recently surrounding the use of thiazolidinediones, which work as 'insulin sensitizers'. In 2007 a meta-analysis was published which demonstrated that those taking rosiglitazone had a significant increase in the risk of myocardial infarction (OR 1.43;$P = 0.03$) and a near significant risk in the risk of death from cardiovascular causes compared with other treatments for type 2 diabetes or placebo [37]. The mean age of recruitment to these studies averaged less than 57 years, much younger than our elderly population, where the cardiovascular risk is much higher. Similarly, these drugs are associated with an increased risk of fluid retention and heart failure. In addition, the risk of fracture at multiple (largely peripheral) sites is doubled in women using rosiglitazone or pioglitazone in the long-term [38], with numbers needed to harm just 21 in postmenopausal women. This has lead to a recommendation by the National Institute for Health and Clinical Excellence (NICE) to stop or not initiate thiazolidinediones in those people 'who have evidence of heart failure or who are at higher risk of fracture' [39]. Most recently, and largely due to the evidence that has accumulated regarding cardiovascular risk, the European Medicines Agency (in addition to the U.S Food and Drug Administration) have taken regulatory action on rosiglitazone to recommend suspension of the marketing authorisations for all rosiglitazone-containing products [40]. In the foreseeable future, the use of this class of drug is surely likely to decrease.

The European Diabetes Working Party guidelines advise that alpha-glucosidase inhibitors (namely acarbose) can be used if other treatments are not tolerated. However, gastro-intestinal side-effects largely limit its use, and it has been largely superseded by newer therapies- incretins. These treatments have a novel mechanism of action. Following the ingestion of food, glucagon-like peptide-1 (GLP-1) and glucose-dependent insulinotropic peptide (GIP) are released from the intestine, stimulating insulin release and inhibiting glucagon secretion. Enzymes including dipeptidyl peptidase-4 (DPP-4) then degrade these incretins. GLP-1 analogues (which require subcutaneous injections, such as exenatide) and DPP-4 inhibitors (such as sitagliptin and vildagliptin) have now been incorporated into NICE guidelines [41]. DPP-4 inhibitors are recommended as add-on therapies to metformin and/or a sulphonylurea if HbA1c remains high, and exenatide can be used if BMI is >35 kg/m^2 or BMI is <35 kg/m^2 and insulin use would be unacceptable. The advantage of incretins in the elderly are the lack of gastro-intestinal side effects, the low risk of hypoglycaemia and weight-neutral (or weight-loss in the case of GLP-1 analogues) effects [42]. In a non-inferiority trial of vildagliptin versus metformin in those with a mean age of 71 years, the DPP-4 inhibitor was associated with a low incidence of hypoglycaemia, improved gastro-intestinal profile and similar glycaemic control [43]. Further trials and experience will be required to determine the long-term safety and acceptability in this new class of drugs in the elderly.

Hypertension

Trends for hypertension prevalence from NHANES study between 1988–1994 and 1999–2004 show an increased prevalence of hypertension for each age group studied: in the age group 60–69 years, hypertension prevalence rose from 49% to 60% between the two surveys; in those aged 70–79 the prevalence increased from 62% to 72%; and in those aged >80 from 69% to 77%. Overall hypertension prevalence rose by 10% between the two surveys [44]. Target BP for those with diabetes was ≤130/80 mmHg, and the percentage aware of their hypertension had increased from 77% in 1988–1994 to 86% in 1999–2004. Treatment had increased from 68% to

83%, and those who met the target BP of ≤130/80 showed a significant increase from 21% to 33% . A history of diabetes was associated with less hypertension control.

A prospectively designed overview of randomised controlled trials (RCTs) of different blood pressure lowering regimens on major cardiovascular events in people with and without diabetes mellitus concluded that treatment using any of the major classes of BP lowering therapy is likely to reduce cardiovascular events such as stroke, coronary heart disease, heart failure and cardiovascular death in people with diabetes [45].

Antihypertensive treatment with indapamide with and without perindopril has been demonstrated to be beneficial in the treatment of patients over 80 years by reducing fatal and non fatal stroke. 3,845 patients with a mean age of 83.6 years and a mean BP sitting of 173/90.8 mmHg were randomised to treatment or control. By 2 years of follow up mean BP sitting was 15.0/6.1 mmHg (SP/DP) lower and active treatment was associated with a 30% reduction in the rate of fatal and non fatal stroke and a 64% reduction in heart failure. A novel finding was the reduction death from any cause (unadjusted hazard ratio (HR) 0.79). Based on this study, a suggested treatment target for BP in this age group was 150/80 [46].

In the ADVANCE trial, a study of 11,140 patients aged at least 55 years (mean age 66 ± 6 years), the efficacy and safety of routine blood pressure lowering with a combination of perindopril-indapamide was assessed [47]. The primary endpoint was composite of major macrovascular and microvascular disease. A subgroup analysis of people aged below 65 years, 65–74 and at least 75 years was assessed. At baseline 61% of those aged 65–74 and 67% of those aged >75 years had a BP > 140/90 mmHg and 29% and 37%, respectively, had a history of macrovascular disease. Active treatment with perindopril-indapamide reduced BP by 5.5/2.2 mmHg in those aged 65–74 and by 6.9/2.3 mmHg in those >75 years. The absolute benefits associated with active treatment were greater in older people, with the number needed to treat to prevent one primary outcome of 71 for those aged 65–74, and 21 for those >75 years. Benefits were demonstrated for major macrovascular disease, cardiovascular death, all-cause death and total renal events. Active treatments were well tolerated in those >75 years. Older people had greater absolute benefits reflecting higher risk.

Recent evidence from the ACCORD study group show no increased benefit for people with type 2 diabetes and high cardiovascular risk in reducing systolic BP from less than 140 mmHg to less than 120 mmHg [48]. There was no reduction in the rate of a composite outcome of fatal and non fatal major cardiovascular events. Similarly a Cochrane review found that aiming for blood pressure targets of less than 140/80 was not beneficial in terms of reduction in morbidity or mortality [49]. There is also evidence to suggest that actually aggressively treating hypertension may be harmful in older patients. All antihypertensives may precipitate orthostatic hypotension, postprandial hypotension, syncope and falls, due to age-related reductions in baroreceptor sensitivity [50]. Elderly people may be more susceptible to the side-effects of antihypertensive treatment, such as constipation with calcium channel blockers, volume depletion with diuretics and delirium with beta-blockers, especially if they are on multiple medications. Additionally, in a prospective observational study of elderly patients with type 2 diabetes, there was an inverse relationship between blood pressure and mortality in those aged over 75 years (median age 80) [51]. A reduction of 10 mmHg in systolic blood pressure, diastolic blood pressure and pulse pressure was associated with a rise in mortality risk of 20%, 26% and 20%, respectively, thereby questioning the appropriateness of aggressive blood pressure targets for the oldest old.

Practical Recommendations

Target BP

- The recommended target BP [52] in older people with diabetes is 130/80 mmHg, but co-morbidity, expected life expectancy and frailty should all be taken into consideration and treatment should be individualised.

- It is important to measure BP both standing and sitting and in both arms.

Choice of Medication

The first choice medication for treatment if no other medical conditions are present is a diuretic [53], but choice of antihypertensive treatment may be influenced by co-morbidity and other treatments. Centrally acting BP drugs should not be used as a monotherapy because of the high incidence of sedation, they may cause constipation and may precipitate or exacerbate depression [50]. Medication should be commenced at the lowest dose and gradually increased, to reduce the risk of side effects.

Lipids

Lipid lowering therapy has been conclusively shown to significantly reduce the incidence of coronary heart disease and other major vascular events [54]. A systematic review [55] of five large randomised controlled trials [4S, WOSCOPS, CARE, AFCAPS and LIPID] looked at effect of statin therapy compared with placebo in participants older than 65 years. The risk reduction of 32% was similar to risk reduction in people under 65 years (31%) of major coronary events (coronary death, non fatal myocardial infarction, silent infarction, or resuscitated cardiac arrest and unstable angina in one trial). In addition to coronary events, statins undoubtedly reduce the risk of ischaemic stroke in those with a history of cerebrovascular disease [56], but may increase the risk of haemorrhagic stroke in those with a history of intracerebral haemorrhage.

Prevention of heart disease in elderly patients at risk of vascular disease was studied in the PROSPER trial which studied more than 5,000 participants aged 70–82 with follow up for 3.2 years [57]. Pravastatin reduced absolute mortality from cardiovascular disease by an absolute risk reduction of

2.1%, but there was no benefit over placebo for elderly women. All cause mortality remained the same. This was because the risk of death from cancer increased (absolute risk increase of 1.7%). Pravastatin did not cause cancer, as determined by a subsequent meta-analysis by the authors. What seems to have happened is that cancer has now substituted for the cause of death in the elderly.

There is clear evidence that statin therapy is effective in older people but there remains a disparity between evidence based medicine and actual clinical practice. There is evidence that older patients with coronary heart disease (CHD) or risk of CHD are under treated [58–60], possibly because of concern about drug interactions and adverse events. There is a combination of physician non-acceptance and patient non-compliance. Although the evidence base is established that statins reduce CHD in the elderly, the evidence of overall benefit is lacking [61].

In a prospective study of 5,344 men mean age 76.9 years followed for 7 years there was no significant association of ischaemic heart disease (IHD) mortality with total cholesterol values in all men. However, within the groups there was a positive association with total cholesterol and low density lipoprotein (LDL) cholesterol for IHD for those men without cardiovascular disease [62]. Interestingly, although ezetimibe is widely used to treat cholesterol levels to target, there is no outcome data to support this approach [63].

Practical Recommendations

- The European Diabetes Working Party for Older People guidelines state that statins should be offered to those with an abnormal lipid profile (classified as total cholesterol of >5 mmol/L, LDL cholesterol >3 mmol/L or triglycerides >2.3 mmol/L) and no history of cardiovascular disease, if their 10-year cardiovascular risk is >15% [35].
- Statins should be offered as secondary prevention for all those with a history of cardiovascular disease.

- Frailty, life expectancy and co-morbidities should be considered before initiating treatment.

Aspirin

A meta-analysis [64] evaluated the benefits and harm of low dose aspirin in people with diabetes and no cardiovascular disease. The authors reviewed 157 studies and analysed 6 of these studies (a total of 10,117 participants). There was no clear benefit derived from aspirin. In particular there was no statistically significant reduction in the risk of major cardiovascular events, cardiovascular mortality or all cause mortality. However, aspirin did reduce the risk of myocardial infarction in men but not women.

Practical Recommendations

- Currently the indication for aspirin use is secondary prevention of myocardial infarction and ischaemic stroke.

In the light of the above meta-analysis and the Medicines and Healthcare products Regulatory Authority (MHRA) guidance, NICE updated their guidance on the use of aspirin, and has advised that it is not licensed for the primary prevention of vascular events [41].

Physical Activity

Older people with diabetes have more co-morbidities than non diabetic subjects and a reduction in physical function. They are more likely to use a mobility aid [65]. There is increasing evidence that physical activity offers benefits in improving metabolic control and mobility. In appropriately screened older adults without diabetes and with a mean age 71.4 years, a supervised aerobic exercise intervention led to weight loss and increased fitness [66]. Another 16 week study on sedentary older people (mean age 76 years) also showed that exercise improved the lipid profile, diastolic blood pressure, BMI and waist circumference [67].

Although exercise with a significant aerobic component may not be tolerated by sedentary older adults, high intensity low volume resistance training might be better suited to this group, increasing muscle mass and glucose uptake in the muscles. High intensity progressive resistance training in older adults with diabetes for 16 weeks improved glycaemic control (HbA1c reduced from 8.7% [72 mmol/mol] to 7.6% [60 mmol/mol]), and reduced the dose of prescribed diabetes medication in 72% of those who exercised compared with a control group [68].

Practical Recommendations

- Older people should be encouraged to be physically active.
- If aerobic exercise is not tolerated, high intensity low volume resistance training is of benefit.

Life Expectancy and Clinical Decision Making

There is a view that single disease models should not be applied to preventive treatments in elderly people [69]. For example, preventive use of statins shows no overall benefit in elderly people as cardiovascular mortality and morbidity are replaced by cancer. This view maintains that clinical decision making in relation to disease prevention has additional responsibility. By preventing a condition and accepting that death is an inevitable outcome, the means of dying may be shifted to a different condition.

Walter and Covinsky suggest that while physicians cannot precisely determine a patient's life expectancy, they can make a reasonable estimate based on the presence or absence of significant illness or disability linked to charts of average life expectancy for that age-sex cohort [70].

Treatment decisions in older adults are often complex as they require an individualised assessment of outcomes associated with various options. Evidence derived from RCTs is growing on therapeutic options available but this evidence may not be relevant to older patients with complex co morbidity. Often these patients are excluded from large trials. Other factors may influence an individual's clinical treatment decision and these might include the desire for aggressive medical treatment or the preference for independent living. An example of this might include the aggressive treatment of hypertension, which may reduce the risk of cardiovascular events in the future but may have a significant impact on falls (by precipitating syncope and orthostatic hypotension) in the short term. Decision making can be supported by various clinical decision making tools but these have not yet been developed to support care in all areas. Most experience has been derived for decision making support in the use of warfarin/aspirin in non valvular atrial fibrillation and even in this well worked up scenario there are still significant gaps in the information that can be presented to support decision making. However this is very important as understanding absolute risk is highly influential in decision making [71].

Older people with diabetes have been found to frame diabetes treatment goals in terms of functional outcomes such as maintaining independence rather than biomedical measures such as HbA1c [72]. In a consultation they have been found to be less assertive, ask fewer questions and be less likely to than younger persons to challenge a physician's authority [73]. Self efficacy refers to one's belief that they can plan and accomplish behaviour change and is affected by experience, perception of others' experiences and persuasion. It affects motivation choices and thoughts. This has been found to be a useful construct for older people with diabetes to improve glycaemic control, but not blood pressure and lipid control. Interventions that target self efficacy and raise it mean that individuals are more likely to start, persist and succeed at behaviour change [74, 75].

Heisler et al. demonstrated that older adults with diabetes had better overall diabetes self management if they were provided with diabetes information and were actively involved in treatment decision making [76].

Conclusion

Older people may have different priorities and preferences for their care and these may strongly impact on their health decisions. Some may wish to maintain independence while others prefer an aggressive approach to treatment and risk reduction.

Intensive treatment of cardiovascular risk factors is more likely to reduce morbidity and mortality than intensive treatment of hyperglycaemia.

Practical Points

- Older people need more time within a consultation to be fully informed about their care and to participate in decision making.
- Decision making in older people with diabetes is complex and other factors other than biomedical goals need to be addressed including co morbidity and life expectancy.
- Cognitive impairment may affect understanding and rationale, and carers or relatives should be involved in the decision-making process.

References

1. Boult C, Dowd B, McCaffrey D, Boult L, Hernandez R, Krulewitch H. Screening elder at for risk of hospital admission. J Am Geriatr Soc 1993: 41:811–817
2. Hornick T, Aron DC. Managing diabetes in the elderly: Go easy, individualise. Cleveland Clinic J Med 2008: 75:70–78
3. Rodriguez A, Muller DC, Engelhardt M, Andres R. Contribution of impaired glucose tolerance in subjects with the metabolic syndrome: Baltimore Longitudinal Study of Aging. Metabolism Clin Exper 2005: 54:542–547
4. Crandall J, Barzilai N. Treatment of diabetes mellitus in older people: oral therapy options. J Am Geriatr Soc 2003: 51:272–274
5. Szoke E, Shrayeff MZ, Messing S et al. Effect of aging on glucose homeostasis. Accelerated deterioration of beta cell function in individuals with impaired glucose tolerance. Diabetes Care 2008: 31: 539–543

6. Chang AM, Halter JB. Aging and insulin secretion. Am J Physiol Endocrinol Metab 2003: 284: E7-12

7. Dale AC, Vatten LJ, Nilsen TI, Midthjell K, Wiseth R. Secular decline in mortality from coronary heart disease in adults with diabetes mellitus: cohort study. BMJ 2008: 337: a236

8. Bethel MA, Sloan FA, BelskyD, Feinglos MN. Longitudinal incidence and prevalence of adverse outcomes of diabetes mellitus in elderly patients. Arch Intern Med 2007: 167:921–927

9. Gerstein HC, Mann JF, Yi Q, Zinman B, Dineen SF, Hoogwerf B, et al. Albuminuria and risk of cardiovascular events, death and heart failure in diabetic and non diabetic individuals. JAMA 2001: 286: 421–426

10. Bertoni AG, Hundley WG, Massing MW, Bonds DE, Burke GL et al. Heart failure prevalence, incidence and mortality in the elderly with diabetes. Diabetes Care 2004: 27:699–703

11. Kronmal RA, Barzilay JI, Smith NL et al. Mortality in pharmacologically treated older adults with diabetes: The Cardiovascular Health Study 1989–2001. PloS Med 2006: 3:e400 DOI 10 1371

12. California Healthcare Foundation/American Geriatrics Society panel on improving care for elders with diabetes. Guidelines for improving the care of older people with diabetes mellitus. JAGS 2003: 51:S265-S280

13. Stratton IM, Adler AI, Neil HAWet al. Association of glycaemia with macrovascular and microvascular complications of type 2 diabetes [UKPDS 35]: a prospective observational study. BMJ 2000: 321:405–412

14. Shorr RI, Franse LV, Resnick HE et al Glycemic control of older adults with type 2 diabetes: Findings from the third National Health and Nutrition Examination Survey, 1988−94. J Am Geriatr Soc 2000: 48:264−267

15. United Kingdom Prospective Diabetes Study [UKPDS] group. Tight blood pressure control and risk of macrovascular and microvascular complications in type 2 diabetes: UKPDS 38. BMJ 1998: 317:707–713

16. Haffner SM, Lehto S, Ronnemaa T et al. Mortality from coronary heart disease in subjects with type 2 diabetes and in non diabetic subjects with and without prior myocardial infarction. N Engl J Med 1998: 339:229–234

17. Curb JD, Pressel SL, Cutler JA et al. Effect of diuretic –based antihypertensive treatment on cardiovascular disease risk in older diabetic patients with isolated hypertension . Systolic Hypertension in the Elderly Program Cooperative Research Group. JAMA 1996: 276:1886–1892

18. Katakura M, Naka M, Kondo T et al. Prospective analysis of mortality, morbidity, and risk factors in elderly diabetic subjects: Nagano study. Diabetes Care 2003: 26:638–644

19. Hubbard RE, Andrew MK, Fallah N, Rockwood K. Comparison of the prognostic importance of diagnosed diabetes, co-morbidity and frailty in older people. Diabetic Med 2010: 27:603–608

20. Rodriguez J, Weiss C, Boyd C, Leff B, Wolff J. A systematic literature review of the trial evidence base for treating diabetes and other chronic conditions in older adults. AGS 2010 S111

21. United Kingdom Prospective Diabetes Study [UKPDS] group. Intensive blood glucose control with sulphonylureas or insulin compared with conventional treatment and risk of complications in patients with type 2 diabetes [UKPDS 33]. Lancet 1998: 352:837–853

22. Holman RR, Paul SJ, Bethel MA, Matthews DR, Neil HAW. 10-year follow-up of intensive glucose control in type 2 diabetes. New Engl J Med 2008: 358:580–591

23. The ADVANCE Collaboration Group. Intensive blood glucose control and vascular outcomes in patients with type 2 diabetes. N Engl J Med 2008: 358: 2560–72

24. The Action to Control Cardiovascular Risk in Diabetes Study Group. Effects of intensive glucose lowering in type 2 diabetes. N Engl J Med 2008: 358: 2545–59

25. Duckworth W, Abraira C, Moritz T et al. Glucose control and vascular complications in veterans with type 2 diabetes. N Engl J Med 2009: 360: 129–139

26. Kagansky N, Levy S, Rimon E et al. Hypoglycaemia as a predictor of mortality in hospitalized elderly patients. Arch Intern Med 2003: 163: 1681–1686

27. Whitmer RA, Karter AJ, Yaffe K et al. Hypoglycaemic episodes and risk of dementia in older patients with type 2 diabetes. JAMA 2009: 301:1565–1572

28. Currie CJ, Peters JR, Tynan A, Evans M, Heine RJ, Bracco OL, Poole CD. Survival as a function of HbA1c in people with type 2 diabetes: a retrospective cohort study. Lancet 2010: 375:481–489

29. Tilling LM, Darawil K, Britton M. Falls as a complication of diabetes mellitus in older people. J Diabetes Complications 2006: 20:158–162

30. Rakel A, Sheehy O, Rahme E, LeLorier J. Osteoporosis among patients with type 1 and type 2 diabetes. Diabetes Metab 2008: 34: 193–205

31. Schwartz A, Vittinghoff E, Sellmeyer DE et al. Diabetes –related complications, glycemic control, and falls in older adults. Diabetes Care 2008: 31:391–396

32. Greenfield S, Billimek J, Pellegrini F, De Berardis G, Nicolucci A, Kaplan S. Comorbidity affects the relationship between glycemic control and cardiovascular outcomes in diabetes. Ann Intern Med 2009: 151:854–860

33. Huang ES, Zhang Q, Gandra N, Marshall H, Chin MD, Meltzer DO. The effect of comorbid illness and functional status on the expected benefits of intensive glucose control in older patients with type 2 diabetes: a decision analysis. Ann Intern Med 2008: 149:11–19

34. National Institute for Health and Clinical Excellence. Type 2 diabetes. The management of type 2 diabetes. NICE clinical guideline 87 May 2009

35. European Diabetes Working Party for Older People. Clinical Guidelines for Type 2 Diabetes Mellitus 2004. Available on: www.instituteofdiabetes.org

36. Papa G, Fedele V, Rezze MR et al. Safety of type 2 diabetes treatment with repaglinide compared with Glibenclamide in elderly people: A randomised, open-label, two-period cross-over trial. Diabetes Care 2006: 29: 1918–1920

37. Nissen SE, Wolsky K. Effect of rosiglitazone on the risk of myocardial infarction and death from cardiovascular causes. N Engl J Med 2007: 356: 2457–2471

38. Yoke YK, Singh S, Furberg CD. Long-term use of Thiazolidinediones and fractures in type 2 diabetes: a meta-analysis. CMAJ 2009: 180: 32–39

39. National Institute for Health and Clinical Excellence. Type 2 Diabetes- Newer Agents (Partial Update of CG66). London: Royal College of Physicians 2009

40. http://www.ema.europa.eu/docs/en_GB/document_library/Press_release/2010/09/WC500096996.pdf

41. NICE and Diabetes: A Summary of Relevant Guidelines. November 2009. NHS Diabetes

42. Abbatecola AM, Maggi S, Paolisso G. New approaches to treating type 2 diabetes in the elderly: role of incretin therapies. Drugs and Aging 2008: 25:913–25

43. Schweizer A, Dejager S, Bosi E. Comparison of vildagliptin and metformin monotherapy in elderly patients with type 2 diabetes: a 24-week, double-blind, randomized trial. Diabetes Obes Metab 2009: 11:804–812

44. Ostchega Y, Dillon CF, Hughes JP, Carroll M, Yoon S. Trends in hypertension prevalence, awareness, treatment and control in older US adults: data from the National Health and Nutrition Survey 1988 to 2004. JAGS 2007: 55:1056–1065

45. Blood pressure lowering treatment trialists' collaboration. Effects of different blood pressure-lowering regimens on major cardiovascular events in individuals with and without diabetes mellitus. Arch Intern Med 2005: 165: 1410–1419

46. Beckett NS, Peters R, Fletcher AE et al. Treatment of hypertension in patients 80 years of age or older. N Engl J Med 2008: 358:1887–1898

47. Ninomiya T, Zoungas S, Neal B, Woodward M, Patel A eta al. Efficacy and safety of routine blood pressure lowering in older patients with diabetes: results from the ADVANCE trial. J Hypertension 2010: 28:1141–1149

48. ACCORD Study Group. Effects of intensive blood pressure control in Type 2 diabetes mellitus. N Engl J Med 2010: 362:1575–1585

49. Arguedas JA, Perez MI, Wright JM. Treatment blood pressure targets for hypertension. Cochrane Database Syst Rev. 2009; CD004349

50. Aronow WS. Treatment of hypertension in the elderly. Geriatrics 2008: 63:21–25

51. Van Hateren KJJ, Landman GWD, Kleefstra N et al. Lower blood pressure associated with higher mortality in elderly diabetic patients (ZODIAC-12). Age Ageing 2010: 39:603–609
52. Chobanian AV, Bakris GL, Black HR et al. The seventh report of the joint national committee on prevention, detection, evaluation and treatment of high blood pressure. The JNC VII report. JAMA 2003: 289:2560–2572
53. Black HR, Davis B, Barzilay J, Nwachuku C, Baimbridge C et al. Metabolic and clinical outcomes in non diabetic individuals with the metabolic syndrome assigned to chlorthalidone, amlodipine, or lisinopril as initial treatment for hypertension. Diabetes Care 2008: 31:353–360
54. Baignent C, Keech A, Kearney PM, Blackwell L et al. Efficacy and safety of cholesterol-lowering treatment: a prospective meta-analysis of data from 90,056 participants in 14 randomised trials of statins. Lancet 2005: 366:1267–1279
55. Bandolier. Statins in older people.http://www.medicine.ox.ac.uk/bandolier/bandb117/bii7-4.html accessed August 2010
56. Vergouwen MD, de Haan RJ, Vermeulen M et al. Statin treatment and the occurrence of haemorrhagic stroke in patients with a history of cerebrovascular disease. Stroke 2008: 39:497–502
57. Shepherd J, Blauw GJ, Murphy MB et al. Pravastatin in elderly individuals at risk of vascular disease [PROSPER]: a randomised controlled trial. Lancet 2002: 360:1623–1630
58. Brekke M, Hunskaar S, Straand J. Antihypertensive and lipid lowering treatment in 70–74 year old individuals –predictors for treatment and blood –pressure control: a population based survey . The Hordal and Health Study [HUSK]. BMC Geriatrics 2006:6:16
59. Safford M, Eaton L, Hawley G et al. Disparities in use of lipid-lowering medications among people with type 2 diabetes mellitus. Arch Intern Med 2003: 163:922–929
60. Chin-Dusting JPF, Dart AM. Age and the treatment gap in the use of statins. Lancet 2003: 361:1925
61. Mungall MM, Gaw A, Shepherd J. Statin therapy in the elderly: does it make good clinical and economic sense? Drugs Aging 2003: 20:263–75
62. Clarke R, Emberson J, Parish S et al. Cholesterol fractions and apolipoproteins as risk factors for heart disease mortality in older men. Arch Intern Med 2007: 167:1373–1378
63. Krumholz H, Hayward R. Shifting views on lipid lowering therapy. BMJ 2010: 341:332–333
64. De Berardis G, Sacco M, Strippoli GFM, Pewllegrini F, Graziano G, Tognoni G, Nicolucci A. Aspirin for primary prevention of cardiovascular events in people with diabetes: meta-analysis of randomised controlled trials. BMJ 2009: 339:b4531
65. Sinclair A, Conroy SP, Bayer AJ. Impact of diabetes on physical function. Diabetes Care 2008: **31**:233–235

66. Finucane FM, Sharp SJ, Purslow LR et al. The effects of aerobic exercise on metabolic risk, insulin sensitivity and intrahepatic lipid in healthy older people from the Hertfordshire Cohort Study: a randomized controlled trial. Diabetologia 2010: **53**:624–631

67. Martins RA, Verissimo MT, Coelho e Silva MJ, Cummings SP, Teixeira AM. Effects of aerobic and a strength –based training on metabolic health indicators in older adults. Lipids in Health and Disease 2010: **9**:76–82

68. Castaneda C, Layne JE, Munoz-Orians L et al. A randomized controlled trial of resistance exercise training to improve glycemic control in older adults with type 2 diabetes. Diabetes Care 2002: **25**:2335–2341

69. Manin D, Sweeney K, Heath I. Preventive health care in elderly people needs rethinking. BMJ 2007: **335**:285–287

70. Walter LC, Covinsky KE. Cancer screening in elderly patients: a framework for individualized decision making . JAMA 2001: **285**:2750–2756

71. Fraenkel L, Fried T. Individualised medical decision making. Arch Intern Med 2010: **170**:566–569

72. Huang ES, Gorawara –Bhat R, Chin MH. Self reported goals of older patients with type 2 diabetes mellitus. J Am Geriatr Soc 2005: **53**:306–311

73. Belcher VN, Fried TR, Agostini JV, Tinetti ME. Views of older adults on patient participation in medication related decision making. J Gen Intern Med 2006: **21**:298–303

74. Trief PM, Teresi JA, Eimicke JP, Shea S, Weinstock RS. Improvement in diabetes self-efficacy and glycaemic control using telemedicine in a sample of older, ethnically diverse individuals who have diabetes: the IDEATel project. Age and Ageing 2009: **38**:219–225

75. Bandura A. Social cognitive theory: an agentic approach. Annu Rev Psychol 2001: **52**: 1–26

76. Heisler M, Cole I, Weir D, Kerr EA, Hayward RA. Does physician communication influence older patients diabetes self –management and glycemic control? Results from the Health and Retirement Study[HRS]. J Gerontology 2007: **62**:1435–1442

Chapter 6
Diabetes and Frailty

Gemma M. Smith and Terry J. Aspray

What is Frailty?

It is apparent that some individuals age more rapidly and become frailer, while others remain robust and physically independent well into their tenth decade. Frailty is a term intuitively understood, but its definition presents a challenge and there is no clear consensus. It is believed to relate to the decrease in physiological reserve and diminished ability to resist stressors, promoting vulnerability in the frail individual. Currently a range of models are used to measure frailty but the choice of components of the model is critical to any definition. Fried and her colleagues incorporate weight loss, self-reported exhaustion, weakness (reflected in poor grip strength), impaired walking speed and low physical activity into their definition of frailty. These criteria are based on normative standards (the lowest population quintile with reference to weakness, walking speed and physical activity) and rather subjective self-reporting of weight loss and exhaustion. They are derived from data from North American populations and have been criticised for their non-generalisability [1], but

T.J. Aspray (✉)
Bone Clinic, Freeman Hospital, Freeman Road,
Newcastle upon Tyne, NE7 7DN, UK

Institute for Ageing and Health, Newcastle University,
Newcastle upon Tyne, NE4 5PL, UK

G. Hawthorne (ed.), *Diabetes Care for the Older Patient*,
DOI 10.1007/978-0-85729-461-6_6,
© Springer-Verlag London Limited 2012

they are well-validated at a population level in the USA. There is always the need to re-validate their use for individuals from other populations and in relation to specific conditions. Rockwood takes an even more epidemiological approach in defining frailty, focusing on the accumulation of *deficits*, which for the most part represent co-morbidities which are associated with an increase likelihood of the presence of frailty, resulting in a vulnerability to impairment [2].

As Abellan van Kan and colleagues point out these two main definitions focus on either a physical phenotype of frailty, based on functional impairments (Fried's criteria) or the multi-domain phenotype, based on a frailty index constructed from the accumulation of identified *deficits* and based on comprehensive geriatric assessment [3]. With the latter, we have a chicken and egg argument of whether the presence of what might be thought of as clinical outcomes of frailty by one definition (for example cognitive impairment) can be reasonably used by the alternative definition as a risk factor for worsening frailty.

The clinical features of frailty (as reflected in Fried's definition) potentially relate to the pathophysiology of diabetes. Weight loss is important when type 2 diabetes and frailty are present. Weight gain is more usually associated with the aetiology of diabetes whereas weight loss is a classic feature of newly diagnosed type 1 diabetes and is often seen at presentation in patients with type 2 diabetes. It is important to regularly monitor weight as weight loss may reflect improvement in glycaemic control and improved insulin sensitivity or on the other hand it can indicate poorer glycaemic control because of relative insulin deficiency typically seen in type 1 diabetes. Moderate weight loss over periods of 4–6 years in older patients with diabetes has little beneficial impact on glycosylated haemoglobin and it is hypothesised that weight loss may reflect disease processes which also result in poor glycemic control [4]. Fried's other criteria, exhaustion and fatigue are common symptoms reported by diabetic patients, particularly those with poor glycaemic control [5]. Decreased walking speed associated with decreased activity is likely to promote a more *diabetogenic* state in those without diabetes and worsen glycaemic control in those with the condition. Finally, muscle weakness, reflecting sarcopoenia, may have an important link with diabetes, as alterations in lean body mass interfere with insulin sensitivity [6].

Whatever the underlying mechanism by which the patient becomes frail, there are challenges presented in managing diabetes for frail house-bound older patients. Moreover, a relatively common outcome in Europe and North America is for frail older people with multiple health problems to reside in care homes. Diabetes has been shown to be associated with an increased risk of admission to nursing homes [7]; and, on screening, at least a fifth of residents of nursing and residential homes have diabetes [8]. The management of diabetes and setting appropriate targets for care for nursing and residential care home residents can be particularly challenging, as these are amongst the frailest of all our patients.

Diabetes and Co-morbidities

Frailty is associated with the presence of a number of co-morbidities. Thus the diabetic patient with cerebrovascular disease, dementia, generalised osteo-arthritis and a previous myocardial infarction is at considerable risk of becoming frail by the time she reaches her ninth decade, if not sooner. Diabetes is an important contributor to frailty in older age, but its relationship with co-morbidities is complex. In some cases, there are direct associations, such as with microvascular disease, macrovascular disease and cardiovascular risk which promote an interaction between the adverse effects of diabetes with a range of conditions, including stroke and ischaemic heart disease. For others, such as the association of diabetes and osteoporosis, the links are not as clear cut.

Vascular Disease

Diabetes is an important determinant of cardiovascular risk. Microvascular disease affects the kidney, peripheral nerves and retina, resulting in nephropathy, neuropathy and retinopathy. The UK Prospective Diabetes Study (UKPDS) confirmed that both hyperglycaemia and raised blood pressure increased the risk of small-vessel disease complications in these patients [9, 10]. With age, these risks continue; but the associated macrovascular risks become increasingly common. Thus ischaemic heart disease and cerebrovascular disease are much commoner in older people with diabetes, with the incidence of stroke 2.5–3.5 times greater than in the background population [11].

The risk of cognitive impairment is also much greater in older people with diabetes. Although an association with vascular dementia is acknowledged, reflecting the increase in macrovascular disease burden, Alzheimer's disease is also commoner in patients with diabetes, as discussed in Chap. 2 (Strachan).

Vascular disease in older frail patients with diabetes may require a combination of primary prevention, secondary prevention and active treatment. In the frailest patients, there are often multiple vascular co-morbidities: for example, peripheral vascular disease, renal impairment and cerebrovascular disease. Blood pressure management to limit disease progression may be influenced by limitations on the risks of adverse effects of a range of antihypertensive agents.

Osteoporosis and Falls

Falls and fractures are important consequences of increasing frailty. Many fractures in older age are associated with falls. One UK study of frail older people found that 86% of fractures were the result of a fall [12]. As recently reviewed [13], there is a complex interaction between diabetes and the risk of falling and fracture and this represents an interesting model of how frailty is associated with multiple co-morbidities. Autonomic dysfunction contributes to the increased risk of falling observed in older people with diabetes. Orthostatic hypotension may be a result of diabetic autonomic neuropathy, side-effects of treatment or, most likely, a combination of both. Commonly prescribed culprit medications given to older patients with diabetes include diuretics, alpha blockers, ACE inhibitors and antidepressants (both tricyclic and newer agents). Drugs with sedative side-effects, such as anti-epileptic drugs used for the treatment of neuropathic pain may also increase the risk of falling.

In addition to postural blood pressure change, gait disorder is a common contributor to falls risk in older frail people [14]. Gait problems in diabetes may be caused by low level neurological disorders affecting the muscles (e.g., diabetic myopathy and statin-induced myositis). Middle level neurological disorders may be due to ischaemic lesions in the posterior cerebral circulation or basal ganglia; and higher level gait disorders involving cortical and subcortical structures may cause gait apraxia, which is commonly linked to cognitive impairment [13].

So we see how frailty in diabetes is linked intimately with the underlying pathophysiology of the condition and causes a range of deficits, each of which is associated with significant impairment in its own right. There are some diabetes-specific mechanisms which are likely to increase the risk of falls and fractures in frail older people. Iatrogenic causes include hypoglycaemia, which is often blamed for unexplained falls in older diabetic patients and hypoglycaemia unawareness can contribute to this [15]. Metformin can (rarely) cause vitamin B_{12} deficiency, which can cause some confusion when teasing out symptoms and signs apparently related to neuropathy. However, low HbA1c, frailty and peripheral neuropathy are associated with an increased risk of falls in older people with diabetes, which suggests the importance of a number of potential mechanisms [16].

Fractures are commoner in patients with diabetes than in non-diabetic subjects and Type 1 diabetes is associated with more than 12 times the risk of fracture. This is probably related to a number of factors, including a low peak bone mass and a tendency for precocious fractures at a relatively young age [17]. Patients with Type 2 diabetes are 1.6 times more likely than people without diabetes to break a bone and 2.8 times more likely to fracture a hip [17]. This is despite the fact that BMD is higher in patients with type 2 diabetes than in non-diabetic subjects. In this case, frailty is probably more important than bone architecture. Finally, frailty in older patients with diabetes is associated with poor vitamin D status and has implications for muscle strength and bone health. The frail older person is less likely to be mobile and to get outside in the summer months, leading to diminished exposure to ultra-violet light for the synthesis of vitamin D in the skin. Poor nutrition may be compounded by the challenge to maintain a diet rich in vitamin D when a low fat diet is promoted to support diabetes management, which may avoid dairy produce and other sources of dietary vitamin D. The result may be that the majority of frail older people with diabetes need vitamin D supplementation (with or without calcium).

Endocrine Disease

There are well recognised links between auto-immune diseases, including type 1 diabetes, coeliac disease, Addison's disease and Graves disease [18]. Moreover, the prevalence of hypothyroidism and hyperthyroidism in the community is increasing [19] and screening for hyperthyroidism and hypothyroidism in older age, whether of auto-immune or other aetiology, has become routine in geriatric medical practice. The clustering of auto-immune and endocrine disorder among older patients with type 1 or (more commonly) type 2 diabetes, contributes to their Rockwood frailty index [2], with important challenges from associated co-morbidity and polypharmacy.

Type 1 Diabetes

The majority of diabetic patients of all ages have type 2 diabetes. New cases of auto-immune diabetes can occur at all ages and after the age of 30 years the incidence of newly diagnosed Type 1 diabetes remains approximately 0.1% per annum for men and women until at least the ninth decade [20]. With improvements in treatment and monitoring of type 1 diabetes, there is an increasing number of older patients who have had type 1 diabetes since childhood or young adulthood, in addition to those presenting at an older age. The presentation of so-called latent auto-immune diabetes of the adult (LADA) can cause diagnostic and therapeutic challenges. In particular, patients who lose considerable amounts of weight and those who have significant ketosis at presentation should be considered for insulin therapy. Lack of insulin reserve, particularly for patients with acute and severe illness, may sometimes be unmasked in some cases where type 2 diabetes had been diagnosed. In older patients with type 1 diabetes the prevalence of the HLA DR3 allele increases although the rate of antibody detection does not [21]. This genetic test is not routinely performed in clinical practice.

In frail older people, specific problems may arise with regard to choice of insulin and its administration. This can affect people in older age with either type 1 or type 2 diabetes where insulin is needed. The simplicity of the regimen, the injection appliance (usually a *pen* device) and its administration, either by the patient or their carer, must be considered. Twice daily injections may be more convenient than a basal bolus regimen, particular when a carer (who may be working) or district nurse is required to give the insulin. If the patient is injecting herself, the appliance must be simple to use and the dial large enough to see when adjusting and administering the dose. It may be difficult for a frail patient or her carer to adjust insulin doses in response to blood glucose readings; but this should be assisted in any way possible and not encumbered by a complex device. With increasing frailty, the loss of body mass and changes in subcutaneous tissue and the skin may be associated with difficulties at injection sites resulting in a failure to rotate location. Repeated injections at the same point may cause local reactions such as lipodystrophy and bruising or injection at sub-optimal sites such as the arms or thighs lead to erratic insulin absorption.

Diabetic keto-acidosis (DKA) may occur at any age in patients with type 1 diabetes. It can present particular problems in older age, where it may not be readily identified, as vomiting is a common presenting symptoms for a range of illness from urinary tract infections to drug intolerance. Unable to give an accurate history, a confused or cognitively impaired patient with Type 1 diabetes may not be identified resulting diagnostic delay. Treatment of acute hyperglycaemia may also be problematic: fluid losses can be exacerbated by adjunctive diuretic therapy for co-morbidities such as cardiac failure. Such co-morbidities also preclude rapid fluid resuscitation for fear of fluid overload and pulmonary oedema. Invasive central venous monitoring may be indicated. Yet, the challenge of ensuring that the frailest of patients gets access to senior medical review, high dependency and critical care is well recognised [22], despite age being an independent risk factor for mortality in DKA [23].

Thyroid

The prevalence of thyroid dysfunction is increased in both Type 1 and Type 2 diabetes and it is helpful to make patients aware of the symptoms, which may be insidious [24]. Hypothyroidism adds to the complications of both diabetes and frailty, causing poor temperature control and tissue quality. Care of pressure areas and the prevention of ulceration may be particularly challenging in patients with thyroid disease, particularly in the presence of diabetic neuropathy. Hyperthyroidism is associated with significant risks of both atrial fibrillation and osteoporosis and, even in its sub-clinical form, the independent contribution of hyperthyroidism to frailty may be significant [25]. Weight loss and diarrhoea associated with thyrotoxicosis may exacerbate an already poor nutritional status. Treatment in frail patients is complicated by significant side effects, including risks associated with symptomatic therapy (such as beta blockers or calcium antagonists). Concerns about the therapeutic administration of radio-iodine are less for older individuals. However, problems are often encountered in exposing carers of reproductive age, their children and/or the staff caring for patients who are resident in care homes. It is important to control hyperthyroidism in frail patients for many reasons. It increases gluconeogenesis and glycogenolysis and so raises serum glucose levels. Hyperthyroidism potentially precipitates impaired glucose tolerance and diabetes and, in those with diabetes, it may worsen glycaemic control and increase insulin clearance by up to 40% [26].

Impact of Frailty on Care

Aims of Treatment

The aim of diabetes treatment in frail older people should be to control symptoms and, where possible, the sequelae of hyperglycaemia. In addition to the commonly recognised microvascular and macrovascular complications already discussed, the frail may be at particular risk of incontinence, recurrent falls, infection, visual impairment, delirium and cognitive decline. More aggressive management to tighten glycaemic control may not confer as much benefit as in younger populations and may predispose to hypoglycaemia. Multiple co-morbidities in frail patients with diabetes complicate management.

Neurological Disorders

Swallowing and motor co-ordination difficulties may prevent patients from administering oral or subcutaneous preparations respectively. Movement disorders with increased involuntary movements may contribute to practical problems with administration of medicines and potentially increase the metabolic rate, increasing the risk of hypoglycaemia.

Cardiovascular/Respiratory Disorders

Poor exercise tolerance and a sedentary state decrease metabolic rate. This can alter demand for insulin or oral medications although this is frequently counter-balanced by a decrease in appetite. The use of steroids in chronic respiratory disease (and other conditions) predisposes to diabetes and will upset glycaemic control in those known to have diabetes.

Gastrointestinal and Nutrition Problems

Impairment of swallowing function, including diminished production and increased retention of oral secretions and difficulties with mouth care occur in older age and with increasing frailty. Oesophageal dysmotility and obstruction may restrict the use of oral anti-diabetic agents. Variable gastric emptying and altered absorption of medicines via the gut wall can affect bioavailability as well as having a direct impact on nutritional status. The main risk for developing gastrointestinal complications from diabetic autonomic dysfunction is the duration of the disease and this may be particularly challenging to treat in older patients, already suffering from nutritional disorders. Weight loss due to a combination of poor dietary intake and muscle loss may alter the therapeutic approach to patients with diabetes. There may be a need to manage the hyperglycaemic effects of nutritional supplements, in the context of immobility and increased metabolic demand from disease processes. At least 20% of nursing home residents are at least 20% underweight [27]. Whereas drug doses in adults are rarely altered to consider their body mass index, the combination of sarcopenia and weight loss may alter the volume of distribution considerably. Poor energy intake leads to further tissue breakdown and hypoglycaemia, which can prove problematic especially in patients with Type 1 diabetes for whom unopposed glycogenolysis should be prevented with regular insulin.

Polypharmacy

The number of daily medications taken increases with age and frailty. This can affect compliance, understanding of medication and predispose to drug interactions. Complications of multiple drug therapies commonly exacerbate the risk of renal dysfunction: in patients treated with metformin, indications for and dosing with ACE-inhibitors and diuretics may need to be reviewed. Meanwhile the metabolism and excretion of all medications used to treat diabetes may alter with the balance of metabolic function of both the kidneys and liver. Glomerular filtration rate (GFR) falls by with age. The effect of this on glycaemic control is multifactorial, with increased renal glucose loss but the accumulation of some anti-diabetic agents (excreted via the kidney) and an increased risk of toxicity. Renal impairment may also affect fluid balance in those with persistent hyperglycaemia and subsequent polyuria.

Tissue Viability

Tissue quality can be severely compromised in those who are frail, immobile, and malnourished. The prevalence of peripheral vascular disease and polyneuropathy in patients with diabetes increases the risk of ulceration and skin breakdown, associated with delayed healing particularly in those without the necessary reserves. Pressure sores develop more quickly in those with diabetes and the risk of infection is higher. The risks are greatest in the old and frail [28].

Sensory Impairment

The prevalence of visual loss increases with age. This may be caused by diabetic retinopathy, cataract or other unrelated disorders such as age related macular degeneration or glaucoma. Visual impairment has a wide range of impacts on diabetes care. It is likely to be associated with a decrease in physical activity and thus contribute to frailty itself. The ability to view a blood sugar monitor, identify medication and administer the correct insulin doses may be diminished and specific aids (such as a glucometer with an audio output) may be required.

Cognitive Impairment

Diabetes as a risk factor for dementia is discussed in Chap. 2 (Strachan). A patient with mild cognitive impairment managing their own condition may begin to forget how to correct a high blood glucose reading or how to manage symptoms of hypoglycaemia. In the early stages the insidious development of cognitive impairment may not be apparent to family members and carers. Education and self management may become increasingly difficult in those with significant cognitive impairment, as the ability to retain and process new information is gradually lost; and as the focus of providing care can fall to a spouse or carer, education must be targeted at them.

Glucose monitoring and adjustments of medication in response to blood glucose levels may be recorded intermittently by patients, carers or by district nurses; but correlation of these results with diet and symptoms (particularly hypoglycaemia) may not be possible in patients with impaired memory who cannot remember their meals or episodes of feeling unwell. Adherence and compliance with medication may become problematic. Are excursions in blood glucose levels because a patient has eaten a high sugar snack or because they forgot their medication that morning? Multiple doses of medication may be administered by accident, precipitating hypoglycaemic episodes. Dosette and Nomad boxes can assist in these situations, as can carer visits for medication prompts. However the need for *meal prompts* may develop when the person with cognitive impairment starts to forgets to cook. Thus, assessment of drug and nutritional adherence are important components in the clinical review of all patients with diabetes, particularly those who are older and frail.

Metabolic demand may differ between older frailer patients. Many with early dementia and physical agility may increase their energy expenditure, often wandering and pacing indoors and outdoors. There may be a change in insulin response, resulting in hypoglycaemic episodes, particular if appetite and nutritional intake decrease. Many frail patients with cognitive impairment will ultimately become sedentary and eventually bed bound with decreased calorie requirements and their therapeutic requirements will need regular review.

Social Aspects

Frail patients are particularly prone to neglect and social isolation, if housebound and unsupported. As frailty progresses, individuals may cook less and fail to get suitably nourishing food, significantly affecting diabetes management. Without a carer or other person responsible for monitoring their needs, it is easy for them to lose access to health care professionals and medications, whether due to a failure to obtain repeat prescriptions or to adhere to the treatment prescribed. Frail patients may be lost to clinic follow up, including foot and eye screening due to difficulties making and attending these appointments. Foot and eye complications of their diabetes become a further risk, contributing to their frailty.

The Importance of Carers

Carers and particularly spouses are very important in supporting patients. They may prompt them to take medications throughout the day, be aware of the early signs of hypoglycaemia, particularly in those patients who suffer from impaired awareness; and they may also liaise with GPs, diabetes specialist nurses and other members of the diabetes team. They often keep a record of appointments and follow up and take charge of meal planning and preparation, as the patient with diabetes (particularly if increasingly frail and/or cognitively impaired) may lack the skills to provide for their own nutritional needs. Carers have a role in vigilance for developing problems, which the patient herself may not be aware of, such as early memory problems or weight loss. There is an excess mortality in older people on losing a spouse [29], even without diabetes as the complicating factor. The loss of a spouse or carer may result in an increased need for home care and in many cases can result in the need for 24-h care in a residential or nursing home.

Despite an increased risk of admission to a care home, many frail older people can be supported in their own house for a considerable time. With increasing frailty, isolation and impaired mobility, the house a person has lived in for many years may fail to accommodate them comfortably. Essential activities of daily living may suffer, resulting in poor self care. For those who cannot mobilise to the kitchen safely or stand for long periods to cook a meal, nutrition may suffer. If access to a toilet cannot be readily gained the risk of urinary incontinence and, in turn, skin damage, may increase. Inaccessibility to bathing or showering may also lead to poor skin condition and an increased risk of infection, especially in the context of chronic skin ulceration. Adaptations within a residence should be sought to allow the person to maintain their independence in their own home for as long as possible and input from the multidisciplinary team, including physiotherapists, occupational therapists and social workers will help to coordinate adaptations to the home and organise the provision of appropriate care to ensure patients are able to stay at home for as long as they can manage.

Care Homes: A Special Case?

Independent living becomes increasingly difficult for the oldest old and many will move into residential and nursing homes as they reach their ninth decade. It is projected that the number of people aged over 85 years will continue to increase from 1.1 to 4.4 million in the next 50 years [30]! Current UK estimates are that there will be doubling of the care home population over this period to more than one million residents by 2050, associated with social and health costs of providing care in excess of £55 billion per annum [31].

Diabetes is known to be an independent risk factor for care home admission [7], and may be present in a quarter or more of care home residents [8]. Care home residents with diabetes are more prone to complications and need specialist input from primary and (in many cases) secondary care. One important aspect is the organisation of services for older people with diabetes in care homes. Patients who have attended hospital diabetes clinical service for many years may find it increasingly difficult to make it to hospital appointments and, particularly for those who are very frail and suffer from cognitive impairment, consultations in the general diabetes clinic may have relatively little to offer. This is where community and GP services are well placed to provide appropriate care with the support of specialist diabetes support from diabetologists or geriatricians with a special interest in diabetes, where appropriate. It is important that care home residents are protected from clinical guidelines derived for working age adults, which may be inappropriately aggressive in their target settings. This has been recognised by Diabetes UK, who have recently published Good Clinical Practice Guidelines for care home residents [32], which present a number of key policy issues, outlined in Table 6.1.

It is important that on-going review is established for older people with diabetes, whether living in their own home or an institution. Identification of the responsible clinician is imperative. Ultimately in the UK the general practitioner has responsibility for ensuring that this is in place, although it may be provided by a range of services from primary or secondary care. Routine care should include monitoring of the feet and eyes, cardiovascular risk, glycaemic control and the avoidance of hypoglycaemia. However, there are specific issues relevant to care home residents which need to be

TABLE 6.1 Diabetes care in Nursing and residential homes – main clinical areas

Clinical issues	Comments
1. Dietary and nutritional policy	Recognition of eating difficulties are important and staff need to be aware of this and of appropriate educational resources.
2. Use of a minimum data set (MDS)	MDS should be agreed between all relevant parties and include most aspects of care outlined in this table.
3. Resident's care plan	Each resident should have an individualised diabetes care plan with agreed objectives including metabolic targets, annual review arrangements, etc.
4. Annual review arrangements	Review should go beyond metabolic parameters alone but include walking ability, balance, mood assessment and cognitive function.
5. Foot care services	Annual assessment for risk of foot ulceration and access to podiatry services are needed.
6. Eye care services	All residents should be considered for retinal eye screening with domiciliary services for those who are immobile.
7. Treatment goal setting	Appropriate metabolic and treatment to be set, avoiding both over-treatment and under-treatment
8. Blood glucose monitoring	blood glucose monitoring is essential and all staff performing this require training
9. Administration of treatments including insulin	Regular review of medication using a care plan is recommended and staff involved in diabetes care should be encouraged to participate in an insulin delegation scheme.
10. Management of infections	Staff should be aware that residents are prone to a range of infections including the skin, respiratory, oropharyngeal, and urinary tract. Prompt assessment and treatment are advised.
11. Patient safety issues	Residents with diabetes are at special risk of a number of adverse events, which include medication errors, hypoglycaemia, and undetected infection. Staff training is very important.

Table 6.1 (continued)

Clinical issues	Comments
12. Vaccination programme	Residents with diabetes should receive timely vaccinations to reduce risk of serious infections. These should include pneumococcal and influenza vaccinations
13. Management of hypoglycaemia	Risk factors for hypoglycaemia should be recognised, including over-treatment with tablets and/or insulin, poor nutrition, renal disease, treatment with multiple drugs, advanced age (>80 years).
14. Referral to hospital	Guidance should be available to promote safe and effective referral and transfer to hospital of residents with acute illness.
15. Quality of care indicators and Audit within the home	The quality of diabetes care can be assessed using a range of outcome procedures, including: • Clinical audit • Use of a MDS • Completion of care plan and review • Implementation of a diabetes care policy
16. Key educational resources	Staff should have ready and easy access to educational resources, including those that are internet-based.

accommodated, not least the potentially massive burden of staff training within nursing and residential homes [33]. These are outlined in Table 6.1.

Summary

In this chapter, we have discussed the links between frailty, multiple co-morbidities and diabetes. We present a brief review of frailty itself, with some key references. It is notable the majority of the evidence base we present for frailty in diabetes comes from epidemiology rather than robust clinical trials, based on interventions to optimise care. This suggests that we are at an early stage in understanding the importance of frailty; but that, with an increasingly aged population, we will need to develop a new evidence base.

We have also focused on some of the less well known links such as the association of diabetes with osteoporosis, risk of falls and fractures. This is clearly an important area for older people with diabetes. We could have also discussed in depth micro-vascular disease, macro-vascular disease and cognitive impairment as other important co-morbidities.

Finally we re-iterate the point that it is inappropriate to apply clinical guidelines developed for young and middle-aged adults with diabetes to a frail population, who did not participate in the clinical trials on which the evidence is based. Collecting trial evidence is likely to be challenging and at present we are left with a number of valuable consensus statements and the experience of clinicians to guide us. We hope that this neglected area of clinical research will produce more evidence of relevance to our ageing and frail population of patients.

Practical Points

- The lack of physiological reserve causing frailty has an important interaction with diabetes
- Exhaustion and fatigue are common symptoms in both frailty and diabetes, presenting diagnostic challenges.
- Multiple co-morbidities and polypharmacy associated with treating diabetes may add to the burden of frailty.
- Diabetic complications and emergencies may present differently in the frail older person.
- Patients' best interests must be the focus of care and reference to appropriate carers and family members is helpful, particularly for patients with cognitive impairment.
- The balance of benefit to harm in treating frail older people needs to be considered, particularly with reference to primary and secondary prevention.
- Care home residents present particular challenges to co-ordinated diabetes care, which are well described in the Diabetes UK *Good Clinical Practice Guidelines*.

References

1. Drey M, Pfeifer K, Sieber CC, Bauer JM. The fried frailty criteria as inclusion criteria for a randomized controlled trial: personal experience and literature review. *Gerontology* 2011;57:11–8.
2. Rockwood K, Mitnitski A. Frailty in relation to the accumulation of deficits. *Journals of Gerontology Series A-Biological Sciences & Medical Sciences* 2007;62:722–7.
3. Abellan van Kan G, Rolland Y, Houles M, Gillette-Guyonnet S, Soto M, Vellas B. The assessment of frailty in older adults. *Clinics in Geriatric Medicine* 2010;26:275–86.
4. Shoff SM, Klein R, Moss SE, Klein BE, Cruickshanks KJ. Weight change and glycemic control in a population-based sample of adults with older-onset diabetes. *Journals of Gerontology Series A-Biological Sciences & Medical Sciences* 1998;53:M27-32.
5. Van der Does FE, De Neeling JN, Snoek FJ, Kostense PJ, Grootenhuis PA, Bouter LM, et al. Symptoms and well-being in relation to glycemic control in type II diabetes. *Diabetes Care* 1996;19:204–10.
6. Morley JE. Diabetes, sarcopenia, and frailty. *Clinics in Geriatric Medicine* 2008;24:455–69.
7. Tsuji I, Whalen S, Finucane TE. Predictors of nursing home placement in community-based long-term care. *Journal of the American Geriatrics Society* 1995;43:761–6.
8. Aspray TJ, Nesbit K, Cassidy TP, Farrow E, Hawthorne G. Diabetes in British nursing and residential homes: a pragmatic screening study. *Diabetes Care* 2006;29:707–8.
9. Tight blood pressure control and risk of macrovascular and microvascular complications in type 2 diabetes: UKPDS 38. UK Prospective Diabetes Study Group. *BMJ* 1998;317:703–13.
10. Effect of intensive blood-glucose control with metformin on complications in overweight patients with type 2 diabetes (UKPDS 34). UK Prospective Diabetes Study (UKPDS) Group. *Lancet* 1998;352:854–65.
11. Kannel WB, McGee DL. Diabetes and cardiovascular risk factors: the Framingham study. *Circulation* 1979;59:8–13.
12. Court-Brown CM, Clement N. Four score years and ten: an analysis of the epidemiology of fractures in the very elderly. *Injury* 2009;40:1111–4.
13. Mayne D, Stout NR, Aspray TJ. Diabetes, falls and fractures. *Age Ageing* 2010;39:522–5.
14. Nordin E, Lindelof N, Rosendahl E, Jensen J, Lundin-Olsson L. Prognostic validity of the Timed Up-and-Go test, a modified Get-Up-and-Go test, staff's global judgement and fall history in evaluating fall risk in residential care facilities. *Age Ageing* 2008;37:442–8.

15. Berlie HD, Garwood CL. Diabetes medications related to an increased risk of falls and fall-related morbidity in the elderly. *Ann Pharmacother* 2010;44:712–7.

16. Nelson JM, Dufraux K, Cook PF. The relationship between glycemic control and falls in older adults. *Journal of the American Geriatrics Society* 2007;55:2041–4.

17. Rakel A, Sheehy O, Rahme E, LeLorier J. Osteoporosis among patients with type 1 and type 2 diabetes. *Diabetes Metab* 2008;34:193–205.

18. Barton SH, Murray JA. Celiac disease and autoimmunity in the gut and elsewhere. *Gastroenterol Clin North Am* 2008;37:411–28, vii.

19. Leese GP, Flynn RV, Jung RT, Macdonald TM, Murphy MJ, Morris AD. Increasing prevalence and incidence of thyroid disease in Tayside, Scotland: the Thyroid Epidemiology Audit and Research Study (TEARS). *Clin Endocrinol (Oxf)* 2008;68:311–6.

20. Molbak AG, Christau B, Marner B, Borch-Johnsen K, Nerup J. Incidence of insulin-dependent diabetes mellitus in age groups over 30 years in Denmark. *Diabet Med* 1994;11:650–5.

21. Kilvert A, Fitzgerald MG, Wright AD, Nattrass M. Clinical characteristics and aetiological classification of insulin-dependent diabetes in the elderly. *Q J Med* 1986;60:865–72.

22. Wilkinson K, Martin IC, Gough MJ, Stewart JAD, Lucas SB, Freeth H, et al. An Age Old Problem- A review of the care received by elderly patients undergoing surgery. London: NCEPOD, 2010.

23. Gerstein HC, Haynes RB. *Evidence-based diabetes care.* Hamilton, Ont. ; London: BC Decker, 2001.

24. Wu P. Thyroid disorders and diabetes. It is common for a person to be affected by both thyroid disease and diabetes. *Diabetes Self Manag* 2007;24:80–2, 85–7.

25. Biondi B, Palmieri EA, Klain M, Schlumberger M, Filetti S, Lombardi G. Subclinical hyperthyroidism: clinical features and treatment options. *Eur J Endocrinol* 2005;152:1–9.

26. Randin JP, Tappy L, Scazziga B, Jequier E, Felber JP. Insulin sensitivity and exogenous insulin clearance in Graves' disease. Measurement by the glucose clamp technique and continuous indirect calorimetry. *Diabetes* 1986;35:178–81.

27. Mooradian AD, Osterweil D, Petrasek D, Morley JE. Diabetes mellitus in elderly nursing home patients. A survey of clinical characteristics and management. *J Am Geriatr Soc* 1988;36:391–6.

28. Slowikowski GC, Funk M. Factors associated with pressure ulcers in patients in a surgical intensive care unit. *J Wound Ostomy Continence Nurs* 2010;37:619–26.

29. Martikainen P, Valkonen T. Mortality after the death of a spouse: rates and causes of death in a large Finnish cohort. *Am J Public Health* 1996;86:1087–93.

30. Wittenberg R, Comas-Herrera A, Pickard L, Hancock R. Future demand for long-term care in the UK: A summary of projections of long-term care finance for older people to 2051. York, UK: The Joseph Rowntree Foundation, 2004.
31. Hirsch D. Paying for long-term care: Moving forward. York, UK: The Joseph Rowntree Foundation, 2006.
32. Diabetes UK. Good clinical practice guidelines for care home residents with diabetes. London: Diabetes UK, 2010:111.
33. Aspray TJ, Nesbit K, Cassidy TP, Hawthorne G. Rapid assessment methods used for health-equity audit: diabetes mellitus among frail British care-home residents. *Public Health* 2006;120:1042–51.

Chapter 7
Perceptions of Users and Carers in Supporting Diabetes Care: Practical Guidance, Support and Information for Carers

Mima Cattan

I am sick of being handed round like a parcel from specialism to specialism. I'm still the same *me* that I always have been, the same *me* that I was yesterday and will be tomorrow.
Margaret Simey, aged 97, (in [1] pp. 26, 28).

Introduction

One of the difficulties older people often face is being treated as bits of chronic health problems, illnesses and illness symptoms instead of being viewed as individuals with the same needs, desires and rights as any other age or service user group. Although diabetes services have improved over the past decade, and recognise that service users and their carers with the right support are able to manage their diabetes,

M. Cattan
School of Health, Community and Education Studies,
Northumbria University, Coach Lane Campus West,
NE7 7XA Newcastle upon Tyne, UK

G. Hawthorne (ed.), *Diabetes Care for the Older Patient*,
DOI 10.1007/978-0-85729-461-6_7,
© Springer-Verlag London Limited 2012

many people with diabetes still report that they do not have a voice in the actual planning of their care [2, 3]. Diabetes is not just a condition of old age but, because type 2 diabetes is more commonly diagnosed in adults over the age of 40, there are particular issues relating to support and care that are more relevant to older people with diabetes and their carers.

This chapter will consider how older people and their carers can be supported to deal with and manage their diabetes. The emphasis is on acknowledging the whole person and the importance of the user – carer relationship in the management of a chronic condition, such as diabetes. The chapter starts by looking at older people's experiences of diagnosis and the specific needs at this transition point. It continues with a section on users' and carers' support needs when living with diabetes, and raises known cultural issues on the subject. It concludes by discussing the potential role of personal budgets [4] in empowering older people with diabetes and their carers to reach a desired level of control over their care planning.

Point of Diagnosis

The most important member of the diabetes management team required to manage the condition successfully is the individual with diabetes [5]. Above all, empathy has been identified as the key in any dialogue intended to support the older person's transition from an acute phase to a continuous person-centred mode of care.

Information Needs – Older People

The diagnosis of diabetes can often come as a shock to the individual, and the response can be anything from anxiety and fear to denial. The Diabetes, Attitudes, Wishes and Needs (DAWN) study, which included 13 countries, found that people frequently lacked even the most basic information about diabetes, including the chronic nature of the condition [5], which would enable them to take informed decisions about their care. Coming to terms with a chronic 'for life' illness can take time (Mosnier-Pudar et al. [6] found negative feelings still persisting after 12 years) and is dependent on good communication with the care providers. Several studies have shown that recently diagnosed individuals and their carers frequently express dissatisfaction regarding communication with their health care providers. Complaints include not having a chance to discuss the questions that are important to them, not being listened to and a feeling of the communication being one-sided [5, 6]. This in turn can create barriers to effective therapy and self management programmes because the information that is given is not timely or personally relevant.

As noted above, at the time of diagnosis, the patient can experience a wide range of emotions, and consequently needs someone who can show them empathy and actively listen to their concerns and questions. They may not be in a fit state to take in a lot of information and advice at that point [5, 7]. Peer advisors have been suggested as a way of supporting health professionals by reinforcing and explaining their health messages and advice and by providing one to one psychosocial support and reassurance to people who have recently been diagnosed with diabetes [7].

When early information, guidance and advice are offered, they should be timely, individually relevant and understandable. Personality traits and perceptions of the health messages given by the physician have been shown to impact on beliefs about treatment effectiveness in newly diagnosed individuals with diabetes [8]. The research suggests that individuals with a high sense of personal and treatment control and greater emotional stability are less likely to attribute their diabetes to psychological causes and more likely to show fewer symptoms and to downplay the consequences of their diabetes. Importantly, however, beliefs about the effectiveness of future therapy seem to be associated with personality characteristics linked to perceptions about how information about diabetes is communicated (fear or reassurance), the amount of information provided and the scope for raising personal concerns [8]. Confusing messages such as the diabetes being 'borderline' or 'mild', or attendance on an education programme being 'voluntary' (and hence not necessary) also impact on the likelihood of attending clinics regularly and adherence to guidance and advice [9]. This illustrates the importance of individually tailoring not just the message itself but also the way the information is communicated.

Information Needs – Carers

Partners and family members as carers have a critical role in supporting older people with diabetes and are therefore an important part of the self-care management team. Yet, frequently carers feel and/or are excluded from discussions about care management [10–12], particularly early on following diagnosis. Carers can have the same feelings of anxiety, confusion and anger as the person they are caring for but in addition, they may feel alone with their worries, responsibility and possible lack of knowledge about the condition, with no one to talk to. The National Service Framework for Diabetes [13] Standard 3: Empowering people with diabetes, includes carers, albeit marginally, as partners in the decision making process about the patient's care. There are potential ethical issues that may arise as a result of such a partnership, and these will be discussed later in the chapter. However, following the diagnosis of diabetes, carers generally can be supported by being included in discussions about the management of the condition, by receiving appropriate information and by having an opportunity to be listened to and to be able to ask questions about what concerns them.

'Trust me! I'm a Patient/Carer' – Living with Diabetes

Older people with diabetes want to be in control of their diabetes. Carers want to be informed so that they can provide appropriate support for the older person they care for. Most research and strategies view patient 'control' as patients being in control of their diabetes through lifestyle changes, blood glucose testing etc., and consequently focus on education, guidance and advice [14]. For example, Mosnier-Pudar et al. [6] highlighted the need for individually tailored education and guidance for older people with diabetes, because although older people were more likely to comply with physician guidance and advice, they were less likely to engage in a bilateral relationship as partners with their physician to plan the management of their diabetes. We could speculate that having a carer present might help to develop such a relationship.

The important question for older people with diabetes and their carers is not simply about controlling the diabetes, but about *retaining control of their lives*. In a focus group (unpublished), older people and carers expressed anger about not being listened to or trusted to take informed decisions about how the diabetes control tasks could be accommodated into their daily lives. Several carers in the group pointed out that lifestyle changes, medication, blood glucose testing associated with the diabetes had to fit within other demands on their time. Echoing the recommendations from the French survey, they wanted information and advice about the management of diabetes that was tailored to their personal circumstances.

Several studies across Europe and elsewhere have found that a major barrier to effective diabetes management for a large proportion of people with diabetes and carers is the lack of knowledge about diabetes or about how to manage it [3, 11, 12, 14]. Worryingly, a substantial number of people with diabetes seem unaware of the seriousness of the condition [14], as illustrated in Fig. 7.1.

In a study in Birmingham, England, of carers providing care for older people with diabetes, the lack of information was one of the main issues raised by the carers. Many provided care without external support and described how they often felt overwhelmed by their caring responsibilities. About two thirds of the carers interviewed provided 20 h or more per week help for the older person and some had been caring

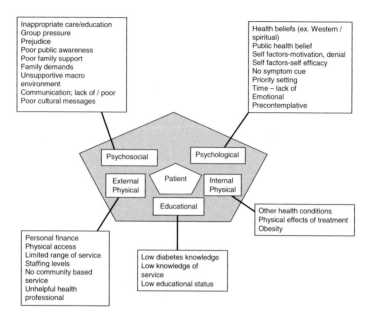

FIGURE 7.1 Barriers to diabetes care (Adapted with permission from Simmons et al. [11])

for over 10 years. The mental and physical strain was significant. In a few cases, the older person received some additional help with domestic tasks. However, none of the carers had been assessed for their needs and many had never received any verbal or written information from a health professional about diabetes and its management. Their main desire was to receive information about local services and sources of support, but their 'wish list' also included practical and regular help with caring, respite care, individual counselling, and the possibility to join a carers' support group.

This experience is mirrored in ethnic minority communities and exacerbated for some by not being able to speak English. In a study in London, carers from South Asian communities expressed frustration over not having the condition explained to them or not, for example, being shown how to inject insulin [15]. Sinclair et al. [12] conclude that feasible and acceptable strategies for diabetes management training for carers are urgently needed. We should bear in mind that in addition to the 'traditional' caring activities, such as personal, medical and general household care, carers can also provide support for the person with diabetes by helping them to modify their diet and to increase their levels of exercise [6].

For many carers the absence of support, advice and information continues over several years. Most carers do not choose to become carers but become carers by default; as partners/spouses, adult children (mainly daughters or daughters-in-law) or close friends or neighbours. Many do not even wish to be defined as *carers*. It would be easy to assume that carers exclude themselves from support and discussions about care management planning as a result of this. This is obviously not the case, as shown above by Sinclair et al. [12] If on the other hand, we look at the various audit, strategy and policy documents dealing with diabetes care [2, 3, 13, 14] it becomes clear that the focus on 'person-centred care', is frequently interpreted as centring only on the patient, with carers mentioned occasionally.

Education and Training

A great deal of attention, in practice and in research, has been given to the training and education for self management strategies to improve clinical, lifestyle and psycho-social outcomes in people with diabetes. Self management has been defined as the active involvement of patients, their family and peers in managing the everyday impact of long-term conditions [16]. Three broad areas have been considered: one to one interaction between the clinician and the patient, didactic education programmes, and patient-centred self management training based on theoretical education (empowerment) models, in particular the therapeutic patient education model. The main differences between a didactic medical model and a person centred model are shown in Table 7.1. Despite a wealth of research, including several in-depth systematic reviews, the

TABLE 7.1 Comparison of medical-centred and person-centred approaches (adapted from Diabetes UK, 2005 p. 21 [18])

Medical-centred model	Person-centred model
Compliance	Autonomy
Adherence	Participation
Planning for patients	Planning with people
Behaviour change	Empowerment
Passive patient	Active individual
Dependence	Independence
Professional determines needs	Individual (patient) determines needs

only thing that seems completely clear is that didactic education does not work [17]. The importance of empathetic, patient-centred communication has also been highlighted [5]. However, it is not clear what components are involved in improving the communication [5, 17], thus making it difficult to determine what changes are needed to improve physician or nurse communication with the patient and the carer.

The purpose of patient education for people with diabetes has been defined as: 'to improve their knowledge, skills and confidence, enabling them to take increasing control of their own condition and integrate effective self-management into their daily lives' [18]. Empowerment and self-efficacy (the belief that it is possible to do something about the 'problem') are key components of patient education programmes.

The Theory

Three main theoretical models have informed the development of therapeutic patient education in diabetes self management:

- The health belief model [19],
- Social cognitive theory (evolved from social learning theory) [20],
- The trans-theoretical, or stages of change, model [21].

The *health belief model* postulates that individuals will take action to protect or promote their health if they:

1. Perceive themselves to be susceptible to a health problem;
2. Believe that the condition can have serious health consequences;
3. Believe that something can be done to reduce their susceptibility or minimise the consequences;
4. Believe that the benefits of taking action will outweigh the costs [19]

The authors acknowledge the limitations of the early model and now include elements of self-efficacy and 'other forces', i.e. social, environmental and economic conditions that influence barriers to action [19, 22].

The *social cognitive theory* consists of six core determinants: knowledge of health risks and the benefits of various health practices; perceived self-efficacy; outcome expectations of costs versus benefits of action; established health goals and ways of achieving them; and perceived facilitators and barriers to change [20]. In addition, it acknowledges through reciprocal determinism, that the individual, their environment and behaviour constantly interact and influence each other [22].

The *trans-theoretical model* is not a true theoretical model, but describes a behavioural change process whereby an individual moves from precontemplation to contemplation, determination/preparation, action and finally maintenance. Relapse is also included in the model and can occur at any point in the behaviour cycle [22].

The Evidence

Evidence from a small systematic review [17] suggests that group-based diabetes education programmes for people with type 2 diabetes can result in clinical improvements and in knowledge about diabetes for up to 12 months. It has also been shown that annual follow-up sessions can maintain the improvement. The findings suggest that group-based education might reduce the requirement for medication, improve self-management skills and increase self-empowerment and quality of life. It would seem that it does not matter who actually delivers the programme, as long as they are trained to deliver a diabetes education programme. As with studies that have investigated one to one physician patient communication it is not clear what precise components of the education programme matter the most. However, it would seem that having face to face contact, a cognitive reframing teaching method and an exercise component in the programme does help to improve glycemic control [23].

Some of the studies in the reviews included carers, but the reviews did not make a distinction between the effects of the programmes on those with diabetes and the carers. This has left Diabetes UK calling for consistent training for carers of people with diabetes (Diabetes UK 2005). They suggest that this training could include the following, adapted to the individual circumstances:

- Insulin and tablet dosage and administration
- The effects of diet, exercise and change of routine on blood glucose levels
- Blood glucose testing – importance and frequency
- Hypoglycaemia awareness and treatment
- Severe hypoglycaemia and Glucagon administration
- How to check the diabetic foot
- Awareness of complications and their symptoms including psychosocial issues
- The need for regular review
- How to access help and support [18]

Recently there has been interest in developing telephone-based education and support for patients with type 2 diabetes. A randomised controlled trial with older diabetes patients, which involved the installation of a home telemedicine unit for blood glucose and blood pressure readings and monthly tele-conferences with a dietician or a nurse demonstrated an improvement in diabetes self-efficacy relating to blood glucose control but not blood pressure [24]. A longitudinal qualitative study, part of a randomised controlled trial, found that a 3 year patient-centred telephone counselling consisted of four overlapping phases: knowledge and perceptions mapping; understanding the person in their own psycho-social context; finding a shared understanding of the patient's problem and its treatment; empowering patients to share responsibility by enabling them to share in decisions they wish to be involved in [25]. It is likely that these stages are similar to the stages in face to face training, even in courses of shorter duration.

The Critique

Therapeutic patient education is not without its critics. To start with, the term 'self management' is contested, with definitions ranging from the possession of biomedical knowledge and skills to psychosocial skills or advocating for better access to services [16, 26]. The main criticism against self management training and structured patient education is in relation to its long-term effectiveness and the lack of cultural, social, economic and environmental considerations. This is particularly relevant in relation to older people, people living in rural communities and ethnic minority communities. It has been said that therapeutic patient education is built on a formulaic framework, which in the main appeals to women, people who are more educated and independent and with ample resources [27]. Older people have over years developed their own idiosyncrasies and established patterns of behaviours and some may therefore find lifestyle changes challenging. In addition, specific issues relating to the ageing process, such as deteriorating eyesight, reduced mobility and multiple health problems may contribute to the difficulties of managing diabetes in later life [28]. Older people in rural areas have the added practical difficulties of accessibility, distance and transport, which limit their ability to attend educational programmes.

What is quite clear from a range of qualitative studies is that older people with diabetes adapt the guidance they receive about the management of their diabetes in line with their personal experiences, norms and beliefs. This is reflected in their decisions about medication and glucose testing, diet, exercise, choosing whether or not to tell others about their condition (the stigma of diabetes) and even about sleep, relating to a fear of falling into a coma [9, 27–29].

Ethical Issues

Although few would disagree that carers should receive sufficient and regular information and support to enable them to continue to provide care for the older person with diabetes, occasionally ethical conflicts may arise that need to be addressed. The most common conflict that occurs is a disagreement between the carer and the older person (mostly spouse/parent/parent-in-law) about the right course of action with regards to medication, diet, and lifestyle generally. The older person may feel that it is their right to take decisions about their own health and that the carer is interfering, while the carer may feel that the older person is at risk (particularly if there is a question of comorbidity and/or cognitive impairment) if he/she does not accept the carer's advice. This is of course not unique to diabetes care, but thought should be given to how it can be resolved. Perhaps it could be included in the Diabetes UK list of training needs for carers as the development of problem solving skills.

Telecare and telehealth initiatives may also raise ethical issues. This was highlighted in a recent study of telecare [30]. Based on the framework originally developed by Beauchamp and Childress [31] the researchers developed the following framework to illustrate the potential problems in the use of telecare:

- **Autonomy** – *the ability of an individual to make choices*
  Autonomy is related to the independence and choice in daily activities that most people take for granted. When people rely on professionals or family carers for their care or for safety monitoring, the introduction of a telecare service can improve or restrict autonomy.

- **Beneficience** – *the principle of working for the benefit of the individual*
  Telecare has the potential to benefit people. It can provide assurance and confidence about their safety and can reduce unwanted dependence on professional staff or family carers. It can also increase comfort through environmental sensors and controls.
- **Non-maleficence** – *the principle of doing no harm*
  While telecare can benefit an individual, it also has the potential to expose people to risk. This is particularly a problem when telecare is used to enhance someone's independence. A balance must be achieved between ensuring safety and invading privacy. The potentially stigmatising effect of telecare, for example wearing a pendant should be recognised and minimised.
- **Justice** – *the moral obligation to act on a fair adjudication between conflicting claims*
  In this case it is about the fairness of resource allocation and access to services. In the interests of justice, resources for telecare services should be allocated so as to balance the needs of the individual with those of the wider community and does not disadvantage one population group at the expense of another (p. 5) [30].

The researchers suggest that these factors should underpin the entire pre- and post- installation process of telecare: assessment; consent; risks associated with telecare use; sourcing equipment (including personalised budgets); installation; privacy; social isolation and well-being; fairness in the allocation of resources.

Cultural Issues

The recognition that cultural factors impact on attendance, acceptance and compliance with self-management programmes has led to attempts to develop education programmes to meet the needs of different cultural groups. Different methods have been used, for example working with community and religious leaders, planning and developing the programme content and materials with community members and continuous community feedback, the use of both written and video recorded materials in appropriate languages and the involvement of community trainers [32]. Contrary to long-held professional beliefs, lack of knowledge is not always the main barrier to behaviour change among ethnic minority groups [33]. Grace [33] found that social norms relating to food and traditional expectations can have a strong influence on how the Bangladeshi community (particularly older people) respond to lifestyle messages.

Serving reduced fat dishes to guests would, for example, be considered inhospitable and shameful by some first generation Bangladeshi adults. In addition, familiar fruit and vegetables may be perceived as expensive, while Western alternatives might not be used because of lack of knowledge about how to prepare them. Exercise opportunities may be restricted for older people because of fear about safety, lack of language skills and because of social norms regarding women's mobility outside the home. An important finding was that although religion was sometimes perceived as a barrier, religious leaders emphasised that healthy lifestyle messages linked to diabetes resonated with the teaching of Islam as part of looking after one's body. The study illustrates that there is a need for culturally relevant health education for ethnic minority older people and carers. It is also important that messages and education approaches are individually tailored to meet the diverse expectations and needs in different age groups and different communities.

A systematic review of health education for type 2 diabetes in ethnic minorities showed that for patient education programmes to be acceptable and useful for ethnic minority groups, simply translating the programme to the relevant language was not sufficient. Teaching and learning styles need to be adapted to the preferences of each community [34]. By having a mixture of approaches, such as one to one and group sessions, the likelihood of health improvement outcomes seems to increase. Unfortunately, because of the small number of studies, it was not possible to tease out if there were any particular issues relating to older people or carers.

A promising form of informal learning through group-based story telling facilitated by bi-lingual advocates has been developed and evaluated in London [26]. The principles of the intervention are based on the notion that communities with a strong oral story telling tradition can increase their knowledge and initiate lifestyle changes through the promotion of story telling. Although the evaluation did not show significant clinically measured improvements, the qualitative evaluation indicated that the group provided opportunities to make sense of their situation and experience, for personalising implicit knowledge, developing social networks, social modelling and critical health literacy. The story telling groups, therefore, provided a rich environment for translating their experiences and knowledge into *how* to manage their diabetes. The authors suggest that to improve and optimise the scope of story telling, the model should be adapted to include individual goal setting and care planning.

Personal Budgets

Personal budgets will come into effect by 2013. A personal budget is defined as:

> The amount of money that will fund a person's care and support costs. It is calculated by assessing a person's needs. It is spent in line with a support plan that has been agreed by both the person and the council. It can be either a full or a partial contribution to such costs. The person may also choose to pay for additional support on top of the budget. So the term personal budget refers to social care money (p. 5) [4].

In principle many agencies, including Diabetes UK and Age UK welcome the concept of older people [with chronic conditions] having control over their care budgets to be able to decide what services are best for them. An evaluation of the first pilot highlighted that older people who received personal budgets did not find the personal budgets easy to use and ended up with lower psychological well-being than other groups, possibly because of the anxiety of 'the additional burden' of being responsible for their own budgets [35]. Some older people did not like the idea of employing their carer. At the time of writing, there are still several questions that remain open, including the issue of the funding of long-term care. In response to Glendinning et al.'s evaluation findings, the Government has published *Putting People First: Personal budgets for older people – making it happen* (2010), for councils and their partners to help in developing increases in older people's choice and control over the care and support they require [4]. The report is intended to eliminate some of the early concerns about the true value of personal budgets and to demonstrate the potential for person-centred approaches in providing flexible, individualised services.

Conclusions

In conclusion, a combination of research evidence and examples of 'promising practice' provide some guidelines on how older people and their carers can be supported in one to one consultations and in group-based, person-centred education. In one to one support, empathy, active listening and allowing time for the older person/carer to ask the questions that matter to them, without dismissing their concerns is central to good patient education. Cultural awareness is critical at this stage. For patient/carer education groups to be effective and acceptable it is important that the framework for the groups has been developed together with the intended population group to identify potential barriers to diabetes self management and acceptable education methods to address the barriers and to support long-term behaviour change. Groups can be facilitated by physicians, nurses, dieticians or lay health trainers as long as they are adequately trained for the purpose. Annual 'refresher sessions' are a way of maintaining and updating lifestyle changes. They can also help to provide long-term psychosocial support for both older people and their carers.

Practical Points

- Empathy, active listening and allowing time for questions that matter to the individual to be asked is central to good patient education when supporting older people and their carers on a one to one basis
- Patient/carer education groups should be developed with the intended population group to ensure that the content is relevant and the methods acceptable to support long-term behaviour change
- Annual refresher sessions can help to maintain lifestyle changes and provide psychosocial support for older people with diabetes and their carers
- Cultural awareness is essential to ensure support and care that is relevant to the individual
- Health professionals should receive appropriate training to support long term behaviour change

In conclusion care and support should be

- Person-centred
- Individually relevant
- Culturally sensitive
- Ethically fair.

References

1. Owen, T., *Dying in Older Age, reflections and experiences from an older person's perspective*. 2005, Help the Aged: London.
2. Audit Commission, *Testing Times. A review of diabetes services in England and Wales*. 2000, The Audit Commission: London.
3. Commission for Health Care Audit and Inspection, *Managing diabetes. Improving services for people with diabetes*. 2007, Commission for Health Care Audit and Inspection: London.
4. Department of Health, *Personal budgets for older people - making it happen*. 2010, DH: London.
5. Skovlund, S. *Diabetes Attitudes, Wishes and Needs*. Diabetes Voice 2004 **49:** 4–11.
6. Mosnier-Pudar, H., Hochberg G, Eschwege E ,Virally M-L, Halimi S et al., *How do patients with type 2 diabetes perceive their disease?*

Insights from the French DIABASIS survey. Diabet Metab 2009. **35**: 220–227.

7. Baksi, A.K., *Experiences in peer-to-peer training in diabetes mellitus: challenges and implications.* Family Practice 2010. **27**: I40-I45.

8. Lawson, V.L., Bundy C, Harvey JN, *The influence of health threat communication and personality traits on personal models of diabetes in newly diagnosed diabetic patients.* Diabet Med 2007. **24**:883–891.

9. Visram, S. Bremner AS, Harrington B E, Hawthorne G. *Factors affecting uptake of an education and physical activity programme for newly diagnosed type 2 diabetes.* Eur Diabetes Nurs 2008. **5**: 17–22.

10. Insulin Dependent Diabetes Trust. *Carers and Diabetes.* 2011 05 January 2011]; Available from: http://www.iddt.org/carers-corner/carers-and-diabetes/.

11. Simmons, D., Voyle JA, Rush E, Dear M. *The New Zealand experience in peer support interventions among people with diabetes.* Family Practice, 2010. **27**: I53-I61.

12. Sinclair, A.J.,Armes DG, Randhawa R, Bayer AJ. *Caring for older adults with diabetes mellitus: characteristics of carers and their prime roles and responsibilities.* Diabet Med 2010. **27**:1055–1059.

13. Department of Health, *National Service Framework for Diabetes.* 2001, DH: London.

14. GfK Health Care, *Choosing to Take Control in Type 2 Diabetes.* 2007, GfK Health Care, Lilly, International Diabetes Federation.

15. Katbamna, S.,Bhatka P, Ahmad W, Baker R, Parker G *Supporting South Asian carers and those they care for: the role of the primary health team.* Br J Gen Pract 2002. **52**: 300–305.

16. Jones, M., Mac Gillivray S, Kroll T, Zohoor A., *How is Self-Care defined in the literature.* 2005.www.sdhi.ac.uk/conference06/Martyn%20.Jonesppt.

17. Deakin,T.A., McShane CE, Cade JE,Williams R. *Group based training for self-management strategies in people with type 2 diabetes mellitus. Cochrane Database of Systematic Reviews.* 2005.Issue 2 Art CD 003417

18. Diabetes UK, *Structured Patient Education in Diabetes. Report from the Patient Education Working Group.* 2005: London.

19. Rosenstock, I.M., Strecher VJ, Becker MH, *Social Learning Theory and the Health Belief Model.* Health Education Quarterly, 1988. **15**: 175–183.

20. Bandura, A., *Health Promotion by Social Cognitive Means.* Health Edu Behav 2004. **31**: 143–164.

21. Prochaska, J.O, Di Clemente CC, *Stages and processes of self change of smoking: toward an integrative model of change.* J Consult Clin Psychol 1983. **51**: 390–395.

22. Nutbeam, D, Harris E, *Theory in a Nutshell.* 2004, Sydney: McGraw-Hill Australia.

23. Ellis, S.E.,Speroff T, Dittus RS, Brown A,Pichert JW et al. *Diabetes patient education: a meta-analysis and meta-regression.* Patient Edu Couns 2004. **52**: 97–105.

24. Trief P.M., Teresi JA, Eimicke J, Shea S, Weinstock R. *Improvement in diabetes self-efficacy and glycaemic control using telemedicine in a sample of older, ethnically diverse individuals who have diabetes: the IDEATel project.* Age Ageing, 2009. **38**: 219–225.

25. Gambling T, Long AF, *The realisation of patient-centred care during a 3-year proactive telephone counselling self-care intervention for diabetes.* Patient Edu Couns 2010. **80**: 219–226.

26. Greenhalgh, T.,Campbell-Richards D, Vijayaghavan S, Collard AP, Malik F et al., *The sharing stories model of diabetes self management education for minority ethnic groups: a pilot randomised controlled trial.* 2009, University College London: London.

27. Danish Centre for Health Technology Assessment, N.B.o.H., *Patient Education – a Health Technology Assessment; summary.* 2009, National Board of Health, Monitoring & Health Technology Assessment: Copenhagen.

28. George, S.R., Thomas SP. *Lived experience of diabetes among older, rural people.* J Adv Nurs 2010. **66**:1092–1100.

29. Collins, M.M., Bradley CP, O'Sullivan T, Perry IJ. *Self-care coping strategies in people with diabetes: a qualitative exploratory study.* BMC Endocr Disord 2009. **9**(6).

30. Perry, J., Beyer S, Francis J, Holmes P. *Ethical issues in the use of telecare.* 2010, Social Care Institute for Excellence: London.

31. Beauchamp, T.L., Childress JF, *Principles of Biomedical Ethics.* 4th ed. 1994, Oxford: Oxford University Press.

32. Jack, L., Liburd L, Spencer T, Airhihenbuwa CO. *Understanding the environmental issues in diabetes self-management education research: a reexamination of 8 studies in community-based settings.* Ann Intern Med 2004. **140**: 964–971.

33. Grace, C. *Nutrition-related health management in a Bangladeshi community.* in *Nutrition and health: cell to community.* 2010. Edinburgh: Nutrition Soc, Scottish Section.

34. Hawthorne, K., Robles Y, Cannings-John R, Edwards AGK *Culturally appropriate health education for type 2 diabetes mellitus in ethnic minority groups (Review).* 2008, The Cochrane Collaboration.

35. Glendinning, C., Challis D, Fernandez JL, Jacobs S, Jones K et al., *Evaluation of the Individual Budgets Pilot Programme, summary report.* 2008 Social Policy Research Unit, University of York: York.

Chapter 8
Management of Elderly People with Diabetes in Primary Care

Tom Coulthard

Introduction

Most people with type 2 diabetes in the UK are identified and managed exclusively in primary care. It wasn't always this way. Fifty years ago, patients with diabetes were largely managed by specialists, but since the 1970s care has gradually shifted to the community [1]. In 1997, a primary care based study in Leicester found that the percentage of patients with diagnosed diabetes who received an annual review in their GP surgery had doubled from 17% to 35% in 5 years, over-taking the number reviewed in secondary care [2]. This trend has continued and today, in my own surgery, nearly two-thirds of the patients with diabetes have had an annual review with us in the last year, far more than those who received one from secondary care.

The growing role of primary care in managing diabetes has been reflected in the primary care literature. For instance, the monthly British Journal of General Practice (the Journal of the Royal College of General Practitioners) published only 10 articles, reviews or editorials primarily about diabetes in the 1990s compared to over 30 in the 2000s, including an entire themed issue in 2008. The same period has also seen

T. Coulthard
General Practitioner, Heaton Medical Centre,
37A Heaton Road, NE6 1TH Newcastle upon Tyne, UK

G. Hawthorne (ed.), *Diabetes Care for the Older Patient*,
DOI 10.1007/978-0-85729-461-6_8,
© Springer-Verlag London Limited 2012

the founding of organisations like the Primary Care Diabetes Europe and the Primary Care Diabetes Society which have associated publications and focus specifically on this area.

Delivering high quality diabetes care in an efficient way is an enormous and increasing challenge for the NHS. The prevalence of diabetes among adults in the UK is now estimated at over 5% of the population and is increasing rapidly. In the 2009/10 financial year, over 35.5 million items were prescribed for the treatment of diabetes in England, representing 7.7% of the total cost of prescribing in primary care, an increase from 5.8% in 2004/5 [3].

Elderly patients with type 2 diabetes make up the majority of patients with diabetes. In my own surgery of 11,500 patients, there are nearly 600 patients with diabetes of whom the majority (60%) have type 2 and are over 65 years of age. There is sometimes a perception among both patients and health care professionals that type 2 diabetes in elderly patients is a 'mild' version of the disease. In fact, the high level of disability and co-morbidities found in this age group may exacerbate the impact of diabetes and make its management more challenging. Many patients have the disease a considerable time before it is identified and already have diabetes complications at diagnosis. Despite this, secondary care tends to focus on specific groups, like pregnant women and young people with diabetes, so older people with diabetes in particular are increasingly being looked after in primary care.

This explosion in the prevalence of type 2 diabetes is undoubtedly the main cause of the growing involvement of primary care in diabetes care in the last 30 years. The same period has also seen a revolution in our understanding of diabetes. Landmark studies have not only demonstrated the importance of good glycaemic control, but have shown the importance of addressing other vascular risk factors and taking a holistic, patient-centred approach to care – aspects which primary care is well placed to address. As the diabetes epidemic develops, specialist services will come under even greater pressure and the trend towards managing diabetes in primary care will continue.

This trend presents many challenges to both individual GPs and practices and to the NHS. GPs and Practice Nurses do not have the in depth knowledge of specialists and can struggle to keep up to date with the latest developments. This emphasises the importance of professional education and maintaining strong links between primary and secondary care. Also, providing diabetes care takes organisation, time and other resources and the motivation to look after patients with diabetes varies widely among individuals and practices.

In this chapter, I will explore as an example how the NHS in England has responded as an organisation, with initiatives like the National Service Framework for Diabetes and the Quality and Outcomes Framework before moving on to look at the challenges from a practice level. In the final section, I will examine the particular issues around providing diabetes care for residential and nursing home residents.

Treating Older People with Diabetes in Primary Care – The English NHS Response

The epidemic in diabetes, especially among older people, has led to an ever increasing role for primary care in the management of diabetes. In recent years, national health policy has developed to meet these challenges and ensure that diabetes care is of a high quality, including the National Service Framework (NSF) and the National Institute for Clinical Excellence (NICE) guidelines.

The NSF for Diabetes consisted of two documents. The first, published in December 2001, set a number of overarching targets, with standards in 12 areas such as preventing diabetes and diabetes in pregnancy. The second was published in early 2003 and outlined a strategy for delivering these standards [4, 5]. Although hailed by some as creating a 'tremendous opportunity' [6], others were concerned that some of the standards were vague and that resources were not identified to allow improvements in care [7].

It is notable that the NSF for Diabetes did not set out any specific standards for older people, unlike other groups such as young people with diabetes or pregnant women. However, an NSF for Older People was also published in 2001. This set standards to try and prevent age discrimination and promote patient centred care in the elderly, although it did not address diabetes specifically [8]. As with the NSF for diabetes, there has been considerable debate as to its content and impact [9–11].

It's one thing for organisations to publish standards and guidelines, but it's another thing to translate these into actual changes in practice and improvements in patient care. The Quality and Outcome Framework (QOF), a system for financially incentivising GP practices for meeting certain targets, has been an important mechanism for trying to change the behaviour of GP practices and improve the management of diabetes and other conditions in primary care. I believe it has had a significant impact on the way GPs manage diabetes so it's worth reviewing its history and the controversy around it in some detail.

Introduced in 2004 as part of a new GP contract, the QOF originally consisted of 146 indicators, grouped into four domains; clinical, organisational, patient experience and additional services. The clinical areas included the commonest chronic diseases such as hypertension, stroke, epilepsy, and mental health as well as diabetes. Since then, the QOF indicators and targets have been changed on a number of occasions, for example, with some points being reallocated in 2006 to new clinical areas including obesity and chronic kidney disease. In terms of diabetes, the lowest HbA1C target was reduced from 7.5% [58 mmol/mol] to 7% [53 mmol/mol] in April 2009. In light of evidence that tight glycaemic control may not benefit older adults with type 2 diabetes and increases risks such as hypoglycaemia, this change caused considerable concern that GPs would be incentivised to pursue inappropriately aggressive management strategies in some older patients [12]. From April 2010, NICE has become involved in reviewing and developing the QOF, publishing a 'menu' of suggested new or altered indicators developed by an advisory committee which in 2010 including relaxing the HbA1C target back to 7.5% [58 mmol/mol] and new tighter blood pressure targets for people with diabetes [13] (Table 8.1).

TABLE 8.1 Quality and outcome framework standard for diabetes, 2009/10 (source: Quality and Outcomes Framework guidance for GMS contract 2009/10: Delivering investment in general practice. NHS employers/BMA, March 2009)

Indicator	Points	Payment stages (%)
Records		
DM 19.The practice can produce a register of all patients aged 17 years and over with diabetes mellitus, which specifies whether the patient has Type 1 or Type 2 diabetes	6	
Ongoing management		
DM 2.The percentage of patients with diabetes whose notes record BMI in the previous 15 months	3	40–90
DM 5. The percentage of patients with diabetes who have a record of HbA1c or equivalent in the previous 15 months	3	40–90
DM 23. The percentage of patients with diabetes in whom the last HbA1c is 7 or less (or equivalent test/reference range depending on local laboratory) in the previous 15 months	17	40–50
DM 24. The percentage of patients with diabetes in whom the last HbA1c is 8 or less (or equivalent test/reference range depending on local laboratory) in the previous 15 months	8	40–70
DM 25. The percentage of patients with diabetes in whom the last HbA1c is 9 or less (or equivalent test/reference range depending on local laboratory) in the previous 15 months	10	40–90
DM 21. The percentage of patients with diabetes who have a record of retinal screening in the previous months	5	40–90
DM 9. The percentage of patients with diabetes with a record of the presence or absence of peripheral pulses in the previous 15 months	3	40–90

(continued)

TABLE 8.1 (continued)

Indicator	Points	Payment stages (%)
DM 10. The percentage of patients with diabetes with a record of neuropathy testing in the previous 15 months	3	40–90
DM 11. The percentage of patients with diabetes who have a record of the blood pressure in the previous 15 months	3	40–90
DM 12. The percentage of patients with diabetes in whom the last blood pressure is 145/85 or less	18	40–60
DM 13. The percentage of patients with diabetes who have a record of micro-albuminuria testing in the previous 15 months (exception reporting for patients with proteinuria)	3	40–90
DM 22. The percentage of patients with diabetes who have a record of estimated glomerular filtration rate (eGFR) or serum creatinine testing in the previous 15 months	3	40–90
DM 15. The percentage of patients with diabetes with a diagnosis of proteinuria or micro-albuminuria who are treated with ACE inhibitors (or A2 antagonists)	3	40–80
DM 16. The percentage of patients with diabetes who have a record of total cholesterol in the previous 15 months	3	40–90
DM 17. The percentage of patients with diabetes whose last measured total cholesterol within the previous 15 months is 5 mmol/l or less	6	40–70
DM 18. The percentage of patients with diabetes who have had influenza immunisation in the preceding 1 September to 31 March	3	40–85

From its inception, the QOF has been highly controversial, with some questioning the ethics of financially incentivising GPs [14]. There is evidence that the QOF has improved diabetes care [15, 16], may offer good value for money [17], and has the potential to reduce health inequalities [18]. In addition, it may been particularly beneficial to older people with diabetes [19, 20], and those with multiple co-morbidities [21]. The data from the QOF is also a valuable resource for audit and research. However, as all these studies are observational, it is hard to know whether the observed changes are actually due to the QOF itself rather than a continuation of the pre-existing trend toward improving quality or the result of other initiatives such as the NSFs. A recent review has argued that overall the evidence remains patchy and inconclusive [22].

There are several other potential criticisms of the QOF. Commonly voiced problems are that the system is vulnerable to 'gaming' and that higher score may simply reflect better data recording rather than actual improvements in patient care [23]. Gaming refers to manipulation of the data in order to improve performance. For example, one paper found a trend towards recording blood pressure measurements just below, rather than just above, the target cut-off [24]. Another issue is that practices are able to 'exception report' patients for reasons such as being on the maximum tolerated therapy, removing them from payment calculations. The idea was that patients, such as a frail elderly person, could be excluded from targets that were inappropriate. However, there has been concern that they are potentially open to abuse and could disguise unmet needs [25, 26].

The choice of indicators has also been controversial, with concern that they are not always evidence based. We have already seen an example with the controversial changes to the HbA1C target. Another would be whether it is appropriate to have one set of targets for people with type 1 and type 2 diabetes when the evidence around these forms of the disease are different. Perhaps an even more serious criticism is that the indicators have focussed on processes and biological targets, generally achieved through drugs, and largely ignored elements of treatment like education, dietary advice and support which we know are so vital to effective treatment.

Treating Older People with Diabetes in Primary Care – Delivering Care in Practices

Managing the increasing population of people with diabetes represents a significant challenge not only to the NHS as a whole, but also to each and every GP surgery. A report by Diabetes UK, a leading diabetes charity, on providing care for people with diabetes in primary care stresses that practices need to focus on all stages of the process. This starts with prevention, both in the general population but particularly in those identified as being at high risk of diabetes, and moves through to diagnosis and ensuring that people who develop diabetes are identified at an early stage. This leads to initial management and treatment, and then initial and on-going education and dietary advice. They advise that this should involve appropriate professionals and use adult learning principles, perhaps involving structured programmes and group formats, but it is also important that GPs, practice nurses and other practice staff become involved and reinforce these messages. The final stage is on-going management with continuing patient focussed care [27].

There are many aspects to providing diabetes care and delivering a complete service involves a wide range of people, from the patients themselves and their friends and families, through to Practice Nurses, GPs and a wide variety of other Health Care Professionals, including hospital specialists, Dieticians, Phlebotomists, Retinal Photographers, Podiatrists and Health Care Assistants to name but a few. While there are obvious advantages for patients in having input from so many different professionals, each with their own skills, there are also dangers – that each will only focus on his or her own area, that no one will take overall responsibility, and that certain aspects of care will slip through the net. A key role of GPs and primary care is to take that responsibility, maintain an overview of the situation and ensure that care is well managed and coordinated (Fig. 8.1).

Primary care teams have developed systems and structures to meet these challenges. These start with a register

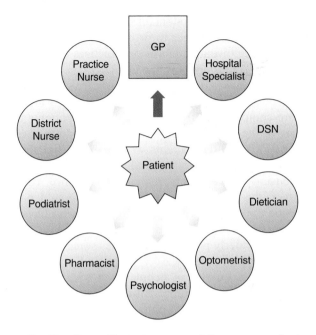

FIGURE 8.1 The figure illustrates some of the many professionals who could be involved in diabetes care. While the patient is always central, the GP plays a key role in coordinating care and taking overall responsibility

of patients with diabetes, an element of the QOF, and a prerequisite to any properly organised service. Most practices have a GP or practice nurse (or both) with a particular interest in diabetes who acts as a clinical lead and keeps his or her skills and knowledge up to date. Many practices have dedicated diabetes clinics and have developed practice guidelines and protocols, often liaising closely with specialist colleagues. A postal survey in 1997 showed that some 96% of practices had a diabetes register and this proportion is likely to have increased still further in the years since then. Two-thirds of practices described themselves as having a 'special interest' in diabetes and more than 70% had a dedicated diabetes clinic [28]. Record keeping in primary care has become increasingly computerised (far more so than in secondary care) which has undoubtedly made it easier to provide an organised service and there is a growing emphasis on practices evaluating the care they provide using tools like audit.

The theory makes delivering diabetes care sound straightforward, but delivering a service on the ground is invariably far more complex and troublesome. Elderly patients represent one of the major reasons why. Not only do they constitute a majority of the patients with diabetes, but the high prevalence of polypharmacy and co-morbidities such as hypertension makes their management more complex. Moreover, this group includes many housebound patients and residential and nursing home residents who have difficulty accessing standard clinics and other services.

The UK's elderly population includes some of the lowest income members of society. According to a European Union report, nearly a quarter of people aged 65 or above were below the poverty line, representing more than two and a quarter million people, with older people being 1.6 times as likely to be below the poverty line than younger adults [29]. As we have seen in the chapter on epidemiology, the risk of diabetes is strongly related to measures of low socioeconomic status with evidence from America also suggesting that low income older people are also at risk of poorer quality diabetes care [30, 31]. The elderly population in the UK is becoming more diverse, with people from a wide range of ethnic backgrounds many of whom may be at higher risk of diabetes than the general population while having greater barriers to accessing healthcare. Practices vary widely in terms of the ethnicity, age profile and affluence of the populations they serve, meaning that the burden of providing treatment will fall disproportionately in certain areas. These facts stress the importance of targeting resources so that the most disadvantaged older people in society can be helped.

A patient of mine illustrates many of the real life practical problems of managing elderly patients with diabetes. Eightyseven years of age, he suffers from a number of medical problems, including chronic kidney disease, heart failure and arthritis, as well as type 2 diabetes. He is effectively housebound and cared for primarily by his wife, a regular attender at the surgery herself with several medical problems of her own, including mental health issues related to the stresses of being a carer and her husband's health. They are increasingly struggling to cope at home, and are currently being assessed for additional support from social services.

His diabetes has historically been poorly controlled and will certainly have contributed some of his other medical problems, such as his ischaemic heart and chronic kidney disease. He was recently started on insulin but he and his wife have struggled to manage his injections and these are now given by the District Nursing team. At one stage he was also seen in secondary care but asked to be looked after entirely by our team as they found the trips to the hospital very difficult and were frustrated at seeing different doctors in the hospital clinic.

For our practice, this case has presented a number of challenges. When I reviewed his notes I noticed that he once went a long time without a diabetes review. Like most practices, our surgery has a well developed diabetes clinic and system for regular reviews. However, as a housebound patient, he was unable to attend the clinic. He was repeatedly invited to the clinic and each time did not attend and was recorded as having simply missed his reviews. He was seen regularly by different doctors on home visits, but these tended to focus on the acute problem rather than his chronic conditions. So, despite having greater needs than most other patients he was actually seen less. Following this and other cases, we have developed a separate system to register patients with diabetes who are unable to attend the surgery so we can make sure they have a regular review and clarify which members of the team are responsible for which actions.

It has been difficult to manage this man's complex mix of conditions and medications. For example, a recent increase in the dose of his diuretics to treat his heart failure caused a deterioration in his renal function. In truth, as a generalist, I have at times felt unsure as to what to do and have needed to consult my secondary care colleagues for advice. They have invariably been very helpful and understanding and this illustrates the importance of using the knowledge of specialist colleagues, even when they do not have primary responsibility for the patient.

The case also illustrates the vital importance of patient education and how this can be particularly challenging for elderly patients. Being housebound, this couple have not been able to access the same range of educational groups as mobile patients and they have found learning new skills difficult. They struggled to learn how to do insulin injections and interpret blood glucose tests themselves and have needed a lot of input from the District Nursing team. Patient education programmes need to recognise the needs of elderly patients and that learning can be intimidating for people who have not undertaken any formal education for many years. At the same time, elderly people often have more life experience which they contribute to help others in a group setting. Research in America indicates that elderly people and their spouses can benefit from diabetes education programmes as much, if not more, than younger people and that support groups in addition to education provide even more benefits [32, 33].

Finally, this case shows the impact of diabetes on the family and carers of sufferers and its potential impact on mental health and how important it is that health professionals take a holistic approach. This is a potential advantage of managing diabetes in primary care as the team is responsible for all aspects of patient care and have knowledge of the wider family and social situation.

Another important issue in managing older people with diabetes is trying to avoid unnecessary acute admissions. Most patients prefer to be in their own home and receive care from their own primary care team. From a wider perspective, this also represents a more efficient use of health resources, freeing hospital beds for other patients. However, as we have seen, older people with diabetes are often frail and suffer from other co-morbidities. This means that they may already be struggling to cope at home so that any acute illness may cause a further reduction in their ability to function and make an acute admission seem like the only safe option. To help prevent this, GPs need to be proactive in identifying people who are struggling and seeing if they can benefit from interventions from team members like occupational therapists and physiotherapist or a package of social care to support them at home. In the NHS in England, the development of community matrons to manage people with chronic diseases in the community has been another practical way of trying to support people in their own home.

From a practical point of view they are many steps that practices can take to try and improve the care they provide to older people with diabetes. These measures are often not complicated and simply require practice team members to be interested and motivated. For example, preventing diabetes by promoting a healthy diet and lifestyle is as vital in older people as for any other section of society and can be especially challenging as retirement and illnesses cause many older people to reduce their level of activity. Educational posters in the practice, individually tailored health promotion during routine health checks, and pointing people in the direction of appropriate activities and groups in the community are all examples of simple yet potentially effective measures that surgeries can take.

In my view, one of the most important practical steps that practices can take is to honestly evaluate their own performance and to critically analyse the root causes where it is poor. For example, it is vital that surgeries have robust systems for detecting diabetes and as the level of undiagnosed diabetes is known to be high, especially in older people. Although I like to think that our surgery provides a high standard of diabetes care, an audit revealed that borderline glucose results were quite often filed as normal rather than having the appropriate repeat tests arranged. We therefore developed a practice protocol, reinforced by an education session and with a copy in every consulting room, which seemed to partially improve the situation. However, a re-audit showed that despite these measures some results were still not appropriately followed up. Talking the problem through with colleagues revealed that we often tried to rush through looking at our results in spare moments between patients. We dedicated to timetable a dedicated slot for reviewing results into surgeries which further improved how we dealt with results.

Diabetes in Care Home Residents

Diabetes in residential and nursing homes is common and treating people effectively in these settings represents a special challenge for primary care. A large survey in the US found that a quarter of nursing home residents aged 65 years or above had diabetes and that people with diabetes were at higher risk of unfavourable outcomes such as emergency department visits [34]. Although the prevalence of diagnosed diabetes has generally been found to be lower in UK studies, at around 10% [35–37], screening studies have found that undiagnosed diabetes is a significant problem with a total prevalence of diabetes of over 20% in residential and nursing homes [36, 37].

Many institutionalised older people suffer from multiple morbidities, far more so than those in the community or in hospital settings. As well as diabetes, dementia, stroke and hypertension are all common in nursing homes, alongside increased risks of acute infections and being admitted to hospital [38]. Many residents suffer from visual and hearing impairment which, together with other problems like impaired cognition, dysphasia and dysarthria, can make communication more difficult. Patients with diabetes often have microvascular or macrovascular complications as well as other conditions like depression and pain and many need extensive help to perform the everyday tasks of daily living [39]. The reduced mobility of many nursing home residents predisposes them to pressure sores and ulcers, problems which of course may be particularly troublesome to people with diabetes.

Polypharmacy is also very common among nursing and residential home residents with diabetes, increasing the possibility of drug interactions and side effects. For example, there has been concern at the high level of prescribing of atypical antipsychotics in institutionalised older people with behavioural or psychotic symptoms [40], drugs which may increase the risk of obesity and affect glucose metabolism [41]. Nutritional problems are a significant problem in nursing homes, including undernutrition and obesity. These problems often involve a number of other factors, such as behavioural problems or disabilities like dysphagia following a stroke, and add to the complexity of providing dietary advice [42].

Although some research suggests that the more structured environment of a nursing home improves diabetes monitoring [43], the quality of care provided is widely recognised as variable and often fails to meet recognised standards, with considerable scope for improvement [44, 45]. In one UK study from the late 1990s, the majority of people with diabetes in nursing homes had no evidence of a review by either primary or secondary care in the previous year and less than a third had had their blood pressure, glycated haemoglobin or renal function checked [35].

Diabetes medications are often not used appropriately in institutionalised older people, with evidence that residents are started on insulin regimens that are inconsistent with guidelines [46]. There is evidence that diabetes medications can be safely reduced in many patients with well controlled blood sugars [47]. Blood glucose monitoring in nursing homes is another area of concern, with concerns that rates of monitoring may be both inappropriately high in some patients but also not frequent enough in others, such as those with possible hypoglycaemic episodes [48, 49]. There have been a number of reports of hepatitis B virus transmission attributable to improper use of monitoring equipment and poor infection control practice both in this country and elsewhere, prompting the Health Protection Agency to publish specific guidance on good practice in this area [50].

We have seen then that older care home residents who suffer with diabetes tend to be more unwell than other people with diabetes, yet suffer worse care. To some extent, the care may be of a worse quality precisely because they are more unwell and therefore inherently more difficult to manage. However, there are undoubtedly other and more complex reasons as well, such as there being various barriers to them accessing the same quality of healthcare that is available to other members of the community.

Often the problem is with communication. We have already discussed how people in residential nursing homes are more likely to have problems in understanding others and getting their message across for at number of reasons. Poor communication between professionals is just as much of an issue. People often enter institutions with poor documentation, such as an incomplete or illegibly scribbled hospital discharge summary. Whether residents come directly from the community or from hospitals or other acute settlings, they will often be registered with a new GP surgery and lose established relationships and structures of care they are familiar with. Also, as more people become involved in providing care, it can become less clear whose job it is to take overall responsibility.

There are also social and physical barriers to care. Family members and friends often act as carers for older people, helping them access healthcare and acting as advocates. Residents of institutions are often more socially isolated than those living in the community and can miss out on this support. Many residential and nursing home residents with diabetes are not able to attend their local surgeries, even with support from staff or family. This means they are unable to access the same services as mobile patients, such as dedicated diabetes clinics in primary or secondary care.

Lack of knowledge and education represent further barriers to care. This is the case with residents themselves, who are less likely to receive the same quality of diabetes education as other people. For example, they are less likely to be able to attend structured education groups like DESMOND, a course for people newly diagnosed with Type 2 diabetes, which are becoming increasing available to other members of the community. Lack of education is also an issue for residential and nursing home staff, who often feel overwhelmed by the complexity of managing diabetes and that they do not have sufficient knowledge and skills. The need for greater education of staff has been noted in a number of studies, with guidelines consistently calling for an increase in training [51, 52].

These factors can mean that institutionalised older people are more likely to miss out on input from different members of the primary care team. We have seen in the section above how high quality diabetes care depends on a diverse multidisciplinary team, with a wide range and number of professionals, and this is particularly true for people who live in institutions because of the complexity of their needs and the fact they are more likely to have or develop complications from their diabetes. For example, the dietary needs of nursing homes residents are often more complicated than those of other people with diabetes and they therefore have even more scope to benefit from the input of a dietician.

There may be another reason why older people with diabetes who live in residential and nursing home do not meet the targets set out in guidelines – that health professionals feel that the targets are not appropriate for some people and decide to ignore them. A recent American study of 11 extended health care facilities found residents were generally well monitored, but despite this few patients achieved treatments goals. For example, blood glucose was monitored in 98%, but only 38% met glucose goals while blood pressure was monitored in 94%, with only just over half meeting the target [53]. While there are many possible reasons for this gap, one possibility is that physicians were deciding themselves that the goals were inappropriately strict in certain patients. This interpretation is supported by a study which asked doctors who care for institutionalised patients how they perceive that they manage patients with different levels of cognitive and functional impairment. Their responses showed that they were significantly less likely to arrange certain aspects of care, such as monitoring lipids or arranging routine ophthalmology, in a patient with functional and cognitive impairment [54].

So is this ageism, with patients being denied proven and effective treatments, or might this represent individualised care, with doctors weighting up all the pros and cons and making decisions to treat conservatively in their patients' best interests? Perhaps there is an element of both. As we have seen above, guidelines for managing diabetes have generally been written for the whole population without at any specific recommendations or treatment goals for older or institutionalised people. Although there are proven benefits to controlling blood sugars and other risk factors, these are likely to be less in older people who at the same time are more prone to side effects such as hypoglycaemia. In certain situations then, it may obviously be appropriate to treat to different targets such as preventing symptoms of hyperglycaemia rather than the standard recommended glucose targets.

On the other hand, I worry that clinicians, care home staff and people with diabetes themselves tend to underestimate both its impact and the potential benefits of treatment. In my own anecdotal experience decisions to treat less aggressively are not usually made in any structured or explicit way, and often without an honest and thorough discussion with the patient and his or her family. Sometimes decisions to treat conservatively are made implicitly because nobody takes responsibility.

Elderly residential and nursing residents with diabetes are clearly a highly vulnerable section of society who face many barriers preventing them from receiving optimum care. Improving this situation will not be easy and will need changes in thinking and behaviour from a wide range of relevant parties from individual clinicians through to the Department of Health. Studies and reviews of this problem have consistently called for specific guidelines, and evidence suggests that nursing homes with specific protocols for diabetes care achieve higher standards than those without [55].

Useful guidelines for managing older care home residents with diabetes were published by Diabetes UK (then the British Diabetic Association) in 1999 and these have been updated [52], with their website also including a section for care home residents themselves and their friends and carers. These guidelines argue that this area needs to be a bigger priority for the NHS and that care home residents should be able to expect their care to be as good as other people's with diabetes.

These guidelines include some practical points that could help GPs improve their management of this group. As these patients have been overlooked historically and are known to generally receive suboptimal care, the potential for improving standards is high. The guidelines call for individualised care plans with clear lines of professional responsibility and improved involvement and co-ordination of the multidisciplinary care team. They recommend that every care home should have a diabetes policy and stress the importance of education for staff. GPs could liaise with their local care homes to find out if these steps are in place. It is advised that practices evaluate the care they currently provide using tools like audit and learning from cases which have gone badly. With a change in culture and measures like these, we can hopefully improve care for this vulnerable group of patients.

Summary

In this chapter we have seen how the diabetes epidemic has led to more and more diabetes care being carried out in primary care, and that this is especially true for older people. This has created enormous challenges, for individual GP practices and the health service more generally, which they are working to meet. At its best, primary care has been able to offer elderly people evidence based and patient centred care delivered by a skilled and diverse multidisciplinary team. We have also explored the unique challenges represented by elderly care home residents with diabetes and how their care might be improved too.

Practical Points

- Primary care is playing an increasingly important role in managing older people with diabetes.
- Being responsible for all aspects of patient care, greater knowledge of the family and social situation, and being easy to access are all potential advantages of care delivered in primary care.
- Older patients with diabetes can be challenging to manage in primary care and issues such as co-morbidities and polypharmacy are common.
- An organised and multidisciplinary approach is essential for providing high quality care.
- Elderly care home residents are at particularly high risk of diabetes and tend to be poorly managed. Greater awareness of the problem and evaluating the level of care currently provided are the first steps to improving standards.

References

1. Kirby M. Review: Fifty years of diabetes management in primary care. Br J Diabetes Vasc Dis 2002;2(6):457–61.
2. Goyder EC, McNally PG, Drucquer M, Spiers N, Botha JL. Shifting of care for diabetes from secondary to primary care, 1990–5: review of general practices. BMJ 1998 1998;316:1505.
3. The NHS Information Centre. Prescribing for Diabetes in England: 2004/05 to 2009/10. London: The Information Centre for Health and Social Care; 2010.
4. The national framework framework for diabetes: Standards. DoH; 2001.
5. The national framework strategy for diabetes: Delivery strategy. DoH; 2003.
6. Young B. The Diabetes National Service Framework - a real opportunity? Clin Med 2004;4:69–71.
7. Greenwood RH, Shaw KM, Winocour P. National service framework for diabetes leaves questions open. BMJ 2003;326(7394):881.
8. The national service framework for older people. DoH; 2001.
9. Morris J, Beaumont D, Oliver D. Decent health care for older people. BMJ 2006;332:1166–8.

10. Evans JG, Tallis RC. A new beginning for care for elderly people? Not if the psychopathology of this National Service Framework gets in the way. BMJ 2001;322:807–8.

11. Manthorpe J, Clough R, Cornes M, Bright L, Moriarty J, Iliffe S. Four years on: The impact of the National Service Framework for Older People on the experiences, expectations and views of older people. Age Ageing 2007;36(5):501–7.

12. Lehman R, Krumholz HM. Tight control of blood glucose in long standing type 2 diabetes. BMJ 2009;338:b800.

13. NICE. About the Quality and Outcomes Framework. http://www.nice.org.uk/aboutnice/qof/qof.jsp [cited 20th October, 2010].

14. Mangin DA, Toop L. The Quality and Outcomes Framework: what have you done to yourselves? Br J Gen Pract 2007;57:435–7.

15. Campbell S, Reeves D, Kontopantelis E, Middleton E, Sibbald B, Roland M. Quality of Primary Care in England with the Introduction of Pay for Performance. New Engl J Med 2007;357:181–90.

16. Oluwatowoju I, Abu E, Wild SH, Byrne CD. Improvements in glycaemic control and cholesterol concentrations associated with the Quality and Outcomes Framework: a regional 2-year audit of diabetes care in the UK. Diabet Med 2010;27:354–9.

17. Walker S, Mason AR, Claxton K, Cookson R, Fenwick E, Fleetcroft R, et al. Value for money and the Quality and Outcomes Framework in primary care in the UK NHS. Br J Gen Pract 2010;60:213–20.

18. Doran T, Fullwood C, Kontopantelis E, Reeves D. Effect of financial incentives on inequalities in the delivery of primary clinical care in England: analysis of clinical activity indicators for the quality and outcomes framework. Lancet 2008;372:728–36.

19. Hamilton FL, Bottle A, Vamos EP, Curcin V, Molokhia M, Majeed A, et al. Impact of a Pay-for-Performance Incentive Scheme on Age, Sex, and Socioeconomic Disparities in Diabetes Management in UK Primary Care. J Ambul Care Manage 2010;33:336–49.

20. McGovern MP, Williams DJ, Hannaford PC, Taylor MW, Lefevre KE, Boroujerdi MA, et al. Introduction of a new incentive and target-based contract for family physicians in the UK: good for older patients with diabetes but less good for women? Diabet Med 2008;25:1083–9.

21. Millett C, Bottle A, Ng A, Curcin V, Molokhia M, Saxena S, et al. Pay for performance and the quality of diabetes management in individuals with and without co-morbid medical conditions. J Roy Soc Med. 2009;102:369–77.

22. Steel N, Willems S. Research learning from the UK Quality and Outcomes Framework: a review of existing research. Qual Prim Care. 2010;18:117–25.

23. Ashworth M, Kordowicz M. Quality and Outcomes Framework: smoke and mirrors? Qual Prim Care 2010;18:127–31.

24. Carey IM, Nightingale CM, DeWilde S, Harris T, Whincup PH, Cook DG. Blood pressure recording bias during a period when the Quality and Outcomes Framework was introduced. J Hum Hypertens 2009;23:764–70.

25. Sigfrid LA, Turner C, Crook D, Ray S. Using the UK primary care Quality and Outcomes Framework to audit health care equity: preliminary data on diabetes management. J Public Health 2006;28:221–5.

26. Roland M. The Quality and Outcomes Framework: too early for a final verdict. Br J Gen Pract 2007;57:525–7.

27. Recommendations for the provision of services in primary care for people with diabetes. London: Diabetes UK; 2005.

28. Pierce M, Agarwal G, Ridout D. A survey of diabetes care in general practice in England and Wales. Br J Gen Pract 2000;50:542–5.

29. Zaidi A, Makovec M, Fuchs M, et al. Poverty of Elderly People in EU25: European Centre for Social Welfare Policy and Research; 2006.

30. Ronny AB, Fabian C, Kelly G, et al. Quality of diabetes care among low-income patients in North Carolina. Am J Prev Med 2001;21: 124–31.

31. McCall DT, Sauaia A, Hamman RF, Reusch JE, Barton P. Are Low-Income Elderly Patients at Risk for Poor Diabetes Care? Diabetes Care 2004;27:1060–5.

32. Gilden J, Hendryx M, Casia C, Singh S. The effectiveness of diabetes education programs for older patients and their spouses. J Am Geriatr Soc 1989;37:1023–30.

33. Gilden J, Hendryx M, Clar S, Casia C, Singh S. Diabetes support groups improve health care of older diabetic patients. J Am Geriatr Soc 1992;40:147–50.

34. Resnick HE, Heineman J, Stone R, Shorr RI. Diabetes in U.S. Nursing Homes, 2004. Diabetes Care 2008;31:287–8.

35. Benbow SJ, Walsh A, Gill Geoffrey V. Diabetes in institutionalised elderly people: a forgotten population? BMJ 1997;314:1868.

36. Aspray TJ, Nesbit K, Cassidy TP, Farrow E, Hawthorne G. Diabetes in British Nursing and Residential Homes. Diabetes Care 2006;29:707–8.

37. Sinclair AJ, Gadsby R, Penfold S, Croxson SCM, Bayer AJ. Prevalence of Diabetes in Care Home Residents. Diabetes Care 2001;24:1066–8.

38. Schram M, Frijters D, van de Lisdonk E, Ploemacher J, de Craen A, de Waal M, et al. Setting and registry characteristics affect the prevalence and nature of multimorbidity in the elderly. J Clin Epidemiol 2008;61:1104–12.

39. Travis S, Buchanan R, Wang S, Kim M. Analyses of Nursing Home Residents With Diabetes at Admission. J Am Med Dir Assoc 2004;5:320–7.

40. Lee PE, Gill SS, Freedman M, Bronskill SE, Hillmer MP, Rochon PA. Atypical antipsychotic drugs in the treatment of behavioural and psychological symptoms of dementia: systematic review. BMJ 2004;329:75.

41. Consensus Development Conference on Antipsychotic Drugs and Obesity and Diabetes. Diabetes Care 2004;27:596–601.

42. Bourdel-Marchasson I. How to Improve Nutritional Support in Geriatric Institutions. J Am Med Dir Assoc;11:13–20.

43. Quinn C, Gruber-Baldini A, Port C, May C, Stuart B, Hebel J, et al. The Role of Nursing Home Admission and Dementia Status on Care for Diabetes Mellitus. J Am Geriatr Soc 2009;57:1628–33.

44. Feldman S, Rosen R, DeStasio J. Status of Diabetes Management in the Nursing Home Setting in 2008: A Retrospective Chart Review and Epidemiology Study of Diabetic Nursing Home Residents and Nursing Home Initiatives in Diabetes Management. J Am Med Dir Assoc 2009;10:354–60.

45. Sinclair AJ, Allard I, Bayer A. Observations of diabetes care in long-term institutional settings with measures of cognitive function and dependency. Diabetes Care 1997;20:778–84.

46. Pandya N, Thompson S, Sambamoorthi U. The Prevalence and Persistence of Sliding Scale Insulin Use Among Newly Admitted Elderly Nursing Home Residents With Diabetes Mellitus. J Am Med Dir Assoc 2008;9:663–9.

47. Sjoblom P, Tengblad A, Lofgren U, Lannering C, Anderberg N, Rosenqvist U, et al. Can diabetes medication be reduced in elderly patients?: An observational study of diabetes drug withdrawal in nursing home patients with tight glycaemic control. Diabetes Res Clin Pr 2008;82:197–202.

48. Gill EA, Corwin PA, Mangin DA, Sutherland MG. Diabetes care in rest homes in Christchurch, New Zealand. Diabet Med 2006;23:1252–6.

49. Aspray T, Nesbit K, Cassidy T, Hawthorne G. Rapid assessment methods used for health-equity audit: Diabetes mellitus among frail British care-home residents. Public Health 2006;120:1042–51.

50. Infection prevention and control guidelines for blood glucose monitoring in care homes. London: HPA; 2009.

51. Sinclair AJ, Turnbull CJ, Croxson SC. Document of diabetes care for residential and nursing homes. Postgrad Med J 1997;73:611–2.

52. Good clinical practice guidelines for care home residents with diabetes. A revision document prepared by a Task and Finish Group of Diabetes UK: Diabetes UK; 2010.

53. Holt RM, Schwartz FL, Shubrook JH. Diabetes Care in Extended-Care Facilities. Diabetes Care 2007;30:1454–8.

54. McNabney M, Pandya N, Iwuagwu C, Patel M, Katz P, James V, et al. Differences in Diabetes Management of Nursing Home Patients Based on Functional and Cognitive Status. J Am Med Dir Assoc 2005;6:375–82.

55. Funnell MM, Herman WH. Diabetes care policies and practices in Michigan nursing homes, 1991. Diabetes Care 1995;18:862–6.

Appendix

HbA$_{1c}$ conversion chart. Older DCCT-aligned (%) and newer IFCC-standardised (mmol/mol) concentrations. Conversions are grouped according to percentage point on the current DCCT-aligned measurement scale. IFCC-standardised values are rounded to the nearest whole number.

G. Hawthorne (ed.), *Diabetes Care for the Older Patient*, 167
DOI 10.1007/978-0-85729-461-6,
© Springer-Verlag London Limited 2012

DCCT (%)	IFCC (mmol/mol)	DCCT (%)	IFCC (mmol/mol)	DCCT (%)	IFCC (mmol/mol)	DCCT (%)	IFCC (mmol/mol)	DCCT (%)	IFCC (mmol/mol)
5.0	31	6.0	42	7.0	53	8.0	64	9.0	75
5.1	32	6.1	43	7.1	54	8.1	65	9.1	76
5.2	33	6.2	44	7.2	55	8.2	66	9.2	77
5.3	34	6.3	45	7.3	56	8.3	67	9.3	78
5.4	36	6.4	46	7.4	57	8.4	68	9.4	79
5.5	37	6.5	48	7.5	58	8.5	69	9.5	80
5.6	38	6.6	49	7.6	60	8.6	70	9.6	81
5.7	39	6.7	50	7.7	61	8.7	72	9.7	83
5.8	40	6.8	51	7.8	62	8.8	73	9.8	84
5.9	41	6.9	52	7.9	63	8.9	74	9.9	85

10		11		12		13		14	
DCCT (%)	IFCC (mmol/mol)	DCCT (%)	IFCC (mmol/mol)	DCCT (%)	IFCC (mmol/mol)	DCCT (%)	IFCC (mmol/mol)	DCCT (%)	IFCC (mmol/mol)
10.0	86	11.0	97	12.0	108	13.0	119	14.0	130
10.1	87	11.1	98	12.1	109	13.1	120	14.1	131
10.2	88	11.2	99	12.2	110	13.2	121	14.2	132
10.3	89	11.3	100	12.3	111	13.3	122	14.3	133
10.4	90	11.4	101	12.4	112	13.4	123	14.4	134
10.5	91	11.5	102	12.5	113	13.5	124	14.5	135
10.6	92	11.6	103	12.6	114	13.6	125	14.6	136
10.7	93	11.7	104	12.7	115	13.7	126	14.7	137
10.8	95	11.8	105	12.8	116	13.8	127	14.8	138
10.9	96	11.9	107	12.9	117	13.9	128	14.9	139

Index

G. Hawthorne (ed.), *Diabetes Care for the Older Patient*,
DOI 10.1007/978-0-85729-461-6,
© Springer-Verlag London Limited 2012